Table of Contents

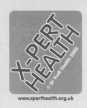

X-PERT Programme - What is it?

Welcome to the award-winning E**X**pert **P**atient **E**ducation versus **R**outine **T**reatment (X-PERT) portfolio of structured education programmes. The X-PERT Diabetes, X-PERT Insulin and X-PERT Prevention of Diabetes (X-POD) Programmes have been developed by Dr Trudi Deakin to help people self-manage their condition, health and quality of life. All the education programmes meet the key criteria identified by the Department of Health, Diabetes UK and the National Institute for Health and Clinical Excellence (NICE).

How will the X-PERT Diabetes Programme benefit me?
You will have the opportunity to explore and address concerns that you may have with your diabetes and learn all about the up-to-date treatments and management of diabetes. There will be the chance to address concerns that you may have with your lifestyle such as your eating plan and physical activity levels and you will be supported in setting your own realistic goals. The aim of X-PERT is not to *tell* you what you should and shouldn't do, but to help you identify what you would like to do and how you would like to do it. The programme can:
- Improve diabetes control by reducing blood glucose levels
- Help you lose weight and reduce your waist size
- Help you identify healthy foods whilst increasing your freedom of choice
- Help you become more active
- Increase your confidence and ability to look after your health
- Improve blood pressure and blood cholesterol levels
- Reduce depression and improve quality of life
- Reduce the medication (tablets/insulin) you have to take for your diabetes

X-PERT Programmes are delivered throughout the UK & Ireland. If you cannot attend a programme or wish to re-cap on the information provided, an interactive DVD programme is available. Visit the public shop on our website at www.xperthealth.org.uk. We hope you find the programme enjoyable and beneficial and welcome your comments. If you would like to share your story or feedback, please email admin@xperthealth.org.uk.

Sign up for the FREE X-PERT newsletter!

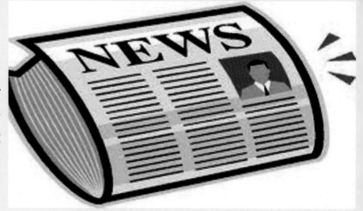

Email admin@xperthealth.org.uk to sign up for the free quarterly X-PERT newsletter. These newsletters provide you with the latest information, useful tips and developments in the treatment and management of diabetes.

X-PERT Health is a charity (registration number: 1143561). Our mission is to enable all people at risk of, or with diagnosed, diabetes to receive good quality structured education that helps them to self-manage their condition leading to improved health and wellbeing.

If you would like to help us with our mission, either by assisting us increase implementation in your area or by making a donation, please visit our website for more information.

X-PERT Programme Summary

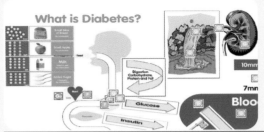

Section 1: What is diabetes?
Digestion, carbs and blood glucose control
The 7 lifestyle factors for optimal health
Health results - what do they mean?
Medications for diabetes
Setting goals: health results

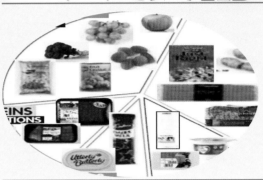

Section 2: Weight management
Energy balance and the Fat Attack DVD
Eating for good health - food groups/portions
Addressing the myths and misconceptions
Physical activity - what, when and how?
Options for weight loss
How to assess what I am eating
Setting goals: eating and activity

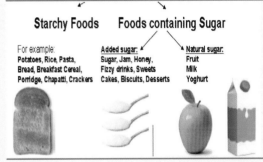

Section 3: Carbohydrate awareness
Carbohydrate and blood glucose levels
Assessing the *amount* of carbohydrate
Considering the *type* of carbohydrate
How good am I at estimating carbs?
What is my daily intake of carbs?
Setting goals: the right carbohydrate for me

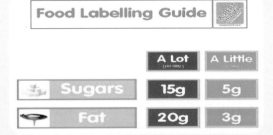

Section 4: Understanding food labels
Fat, saturated fat, sugar and fibre - identifying
"A lot" and "A Little" per portion
The traffic light system
Guideline daily amounts (GDAs)
Nutritional claims - what do they mean?
Setting goals: the foods I buy

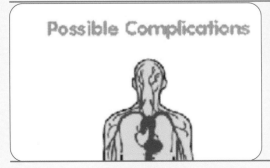

Section 5: Possible complications
Low and high blood glucose levels
How could diabetes affect my long-term health?
Prevention of complications
Importance of regular check ups
Work, driving, insurance, travel and sick days
Setting goals: to reduce risk

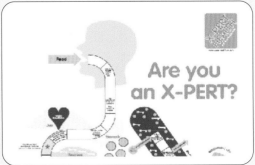

Section 6: Leave the best to the last!
Recapping with the X-PERT Game
What resources are available to help me?
Revisiting my diabetes health profile
Have my needs been addressed?
More confidence to self-manage my diabetes?
Setting goals: self-management in the future...

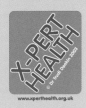

Section 1: What is Diabetes?

Exploring Diabetes

Diabetes is a common condition in which the amount of glucose in the blood at diagnosis is too high because the body cannot use the glucose as energy. Diabetes occurs when the body does not produce enough insulin, or produces insulin but cannot use it properly. There are two types of diabetes:

○ Type 1 diabetes occurs when there is a severe lack of insulin in the body because the cells in the pancreas that produce it have been destroyed. This type of diabetes usually appears in people under the age of 40, often in childhood, and is treated with insulin injections, diet and physical activity.

○ Type 2 diabetes develops when the body can still make some insulin, but not enough for its needs, or when the insulin that is produced does not work properly (known as insulin resistance). This type of diabetes usually appears in people over the age of 40 but increasingly it is appearing in children and young adults. The cornerstone of treatment for Type 2 diabetes is lifestyle changes (dietary changes, physical activity and if necessary, weight loss) but with time, people may also need tablets and/or insulin.

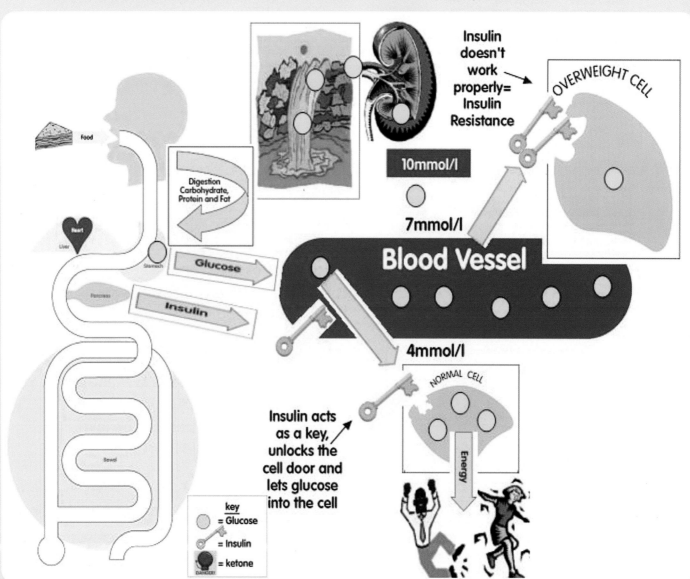

Digestion, Carbs and Blood Glucose Control

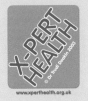

A healthy body needs 6 essential nutrients for life. These are carbohydrate, fat, protein, vitamins, minerals and water. Too much or too little of any of these essentials may not be good for the body. Carbohydrate is the only nutrient that digests and breaks down into glucose and therefore it is the only nutrient that directly affects blood glucose levels. All foods and drinks that contain carbohydrate break down into glucose. The glucose enters the blood.

Glucose is the preferred source of energy for the body but it cannot be used for energy until it enters the body cell. Normally, a person's pancreas (an organ in the body) produces a hormone called insulin, which acts like a key, unlocking the door into the body cell allowing the glucose to pass through into the cell and be converted into energy.

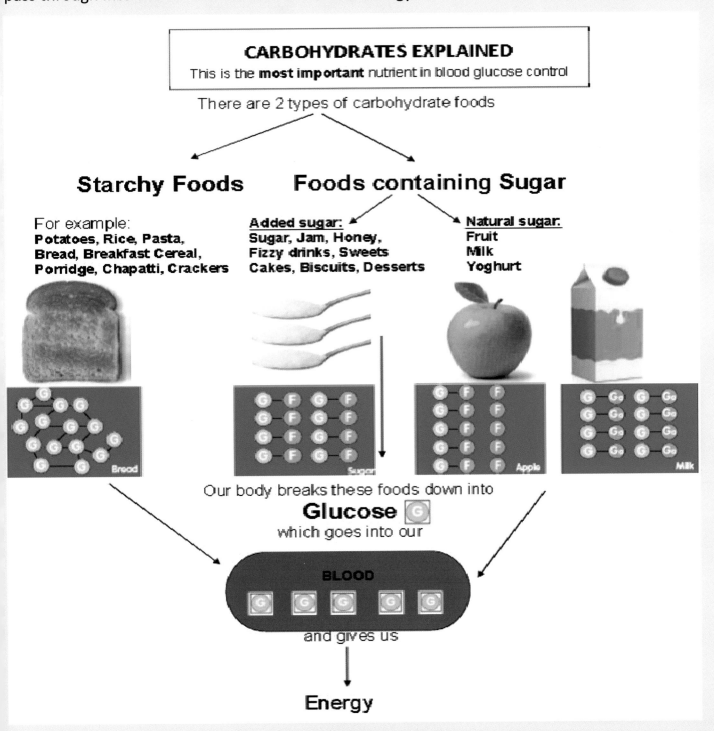

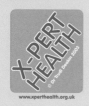

Sources of Carbohydrate Food

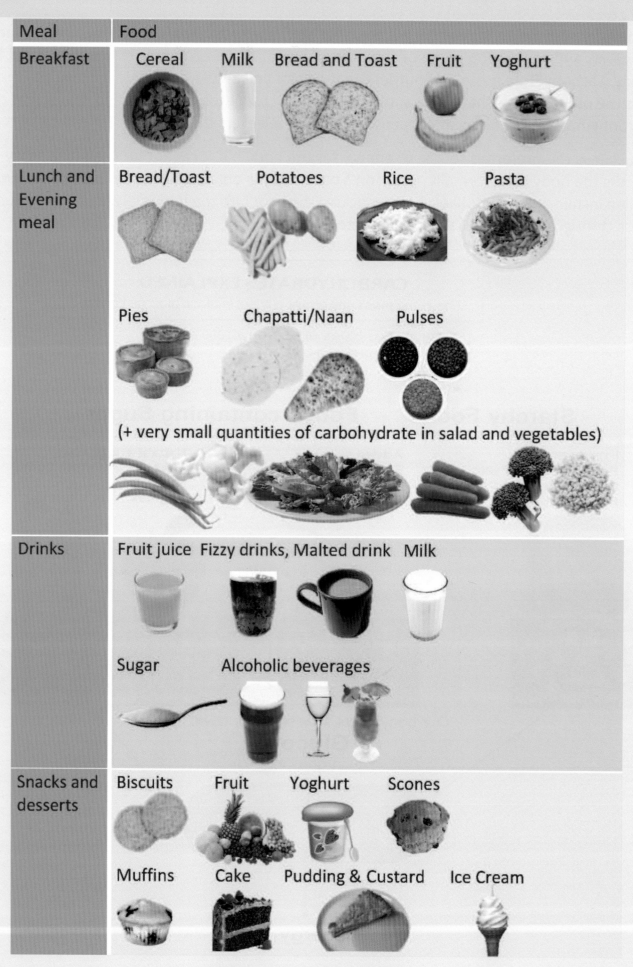

Meal	Food
Breakfast	Cereal Milk Bread and Toast Fruit Yoghurt
Lunch and Evening meal	Bread/Toast Potatoes Rice Pasta

Pies   Chapatti/Naan   Pulses

(+ very small quantities of carbohydrate in salad and vegetables) |
| Drinks | Fruit juice   Fizzy drinks, Malted drink   Milk

Sugar   Alcoholic beverages |
| Snacks and desserts | Biscuits   Fruit   Yoghurt   Scones

Muffins   Cake   Pudding & Custard   Ice Cream |

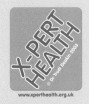

7 Lifestyle Factors for Optimal Health

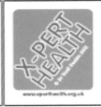

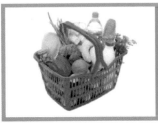

Eating a Healthy Diet

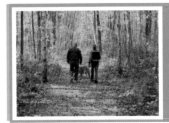

Undertaking Physical Activity

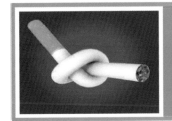

Stopping or Reducing Smoking

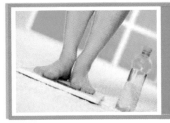

Achieving or Maintaining a Healthy Weight

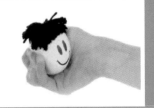

Learning to Manage Stress and Sleep Well

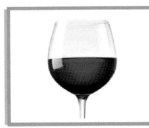

Drinking Alcohol in Moderation

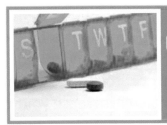

Remembering to take Prescribed Medication

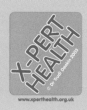

Diabetes Health Profile

The diabetes health profile form (page 82/83) shows you the main health results that your diabetes care team (such as doctor, nurse, dietitian, podiatrist, pharmacist) take into consideration when they monitor your diabetes. If you know and understand what your health results are it may help you to self-manage your diabetes. Ask your diabetes care team for your health results and complete the Diabetes Health Profile form. Remember, the results are *your* health results!

If you have specific questions regarding your own health profile, write them down and discuss these with your diabetes care team during subsequent visits.

Diabetes Health Profile		What does it mean?
Height [m]		Height is measurement of how tall you are. It is usually measured in metres and centimetres.
Weight [Kg]		Weight is measurement of your body weight in kilograms. If overweight, there are major health benefits from losing even a small amount of weight. Excess weight also makes it hard for your body to use insulin properly [insulin resistance] and therefore losing weight helps you to control blood glucose levels.
BMI [Kg/m²] [weight for height calculation]		Body Mass Index [BMI] is an assessment of your weight for height and gives you an indication of whether you are underweight, normal weight, overweight or obese.
Waist Size [cm]		Waist size is a measurement midway between the lower rib and hip bone. If you gain weight around your middle, it will become harder to control blood glucose levels and it will increase your risk of developing heart disease.

www.xperthealth.org.uk

Diabetes Health Profile

Diabetes Health Profile		What does it mean?
Blood Glucose [mmol/l]	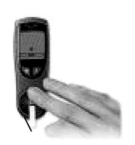	Blood glucose tests give an indication of the amount of glucose in the blood, but only at the time when the blood sample is taken. It involves pricking the finger and placing a drop of blood on a test strip. The blood is then analysed by the glucose meter.
Glycated Haemoglobin "HbA1c" [mmol/mol*]	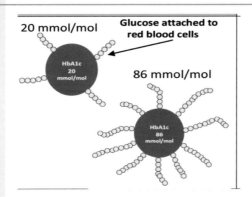	This blood test measures the amount of glucose that is being carried by the red blood cells in the body. It indicates the *average level of glucose in your blood over the last 2 to 3 months.* It is the most important tool to help you and your diabetes care team understand how well your diabetes is controlled. A sample is taken from the vein in your arm and sent to a laboratory to be analysed.
Blood Pressure "BP" [mmHg]	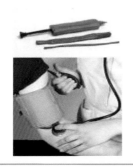	Blood Pressure is the amount of force your blood exerts against the walls of your blood vessels. The first and larger number [systolic BP] is the pressure when the heart pumps the blood into the vessel. The second and smaller number [diastolic BP] is the pressure when the heart is at rest.
Total Cholesterol [mmol/l]	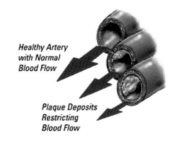	Cholesterol is a fat, which is present in our blood. People with diabetes have a greater risk of raised cholesterol levels. This is caused either by the body itself making too much cholesterol and/or an excess intake of animal [saturated] fat.
HDL Cholesterol [mmol/l] [good cholesterol]	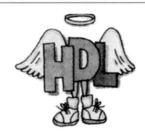	HDL cholesterol is good cholesterol that helps to clear the blood of bad [LDL] cholesterol. The levels of HDL may be increased by regular physical activity and a small quantity of alcohol [less or equal to 1 unit/day] Remember "H" for Healthy!

*The method of reporting HbA1c has changed from percentage [%] to mmol/mol [see conversion table on the back page or calculator at http://www.diabetes.org.uk]

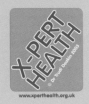

Diabetes Health Profile

Diabetes Health Profile	What does it mean?
LDL Cholesterol [mmol/l] [bad cholesterol]	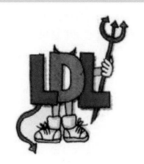 LDL cholesterol is bad cholesterol that encourages a build up of fatty deposits on the lining of the blood vessels. This increases the risk of blockages leading to heart disease and strokes. LDL may be decreased by reducing intake of saturated [animal] fat, increasing soluble fibre and obtaining a healthy weight. Remember "L" for lethal!
Triglycerides (mmol/l)	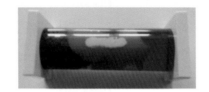 Triglycerides are the end product of breaking down fats in food. Some are made in the body from carbohydrates. High levels have been linked to heart disease. You can reduce levels by being active, eating oily fish and reducing total calories and alcohol intake.
Kidney Function Tests Albumin to creatinine ratio [ACR] Estimated glomerular filtration rate [eGRF]	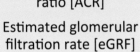 The kidneys filter the blood, removing waste and water to make urine. Tests check how well the kidneys are functioning. The ACR test assesses whether too much protein is leaking into the urine and the eGFR test measures how much blood the kidneys are filtering.
Prescribed Diabetes Medication	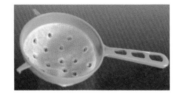 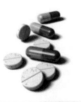 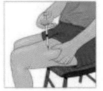 More detailed information about the main types of diabetes medication can be found on pages 74 to 81)	Diabetes medication is needed if blood glucose levels are not controlled with dietary changes and physical activity.* **Metformin:** improves insulin action and reduces glucose release from the liver. **Acarbose:** slows carb digestion . **Sulphonylurea:** stimulates the pancreas to make more insulin. **Prandial glucose regulator:** rapid stimulation of the pancreas and shorter acting reducing risk of hypos. **Glitazone:** reduces insulin resistance. **Incretin mimetic** (injectable): acts like a natural occurring gut hormone that controls blood glucose. **DPP-4 Inhibitor:** allows the gut hormone to carry on working for longer. **SGLT2 inhibitor:** removes excess glucose from the body in the urine. **Insulin:** Injectable. There are different insulins with varying speeds of action.

*Changing diet and/or activity levels may be all that is required to improve blood glucose levels.

Are you a Healthy Weight?

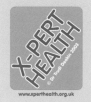

Use the chart below to check if you are a healthy weight. Find your height and draw a horizontal line across and then find your weight and draw a vertical line. Where the two lines meet will show you what weight section you are in. The World Health Organisation has published different BMI thresholds for Asian people as evidence suggests that people from black, Asian and other minority ethnic groups are at a higher risk of diabetes and other health conditions at a lower body mass index (BMI) than white populations.

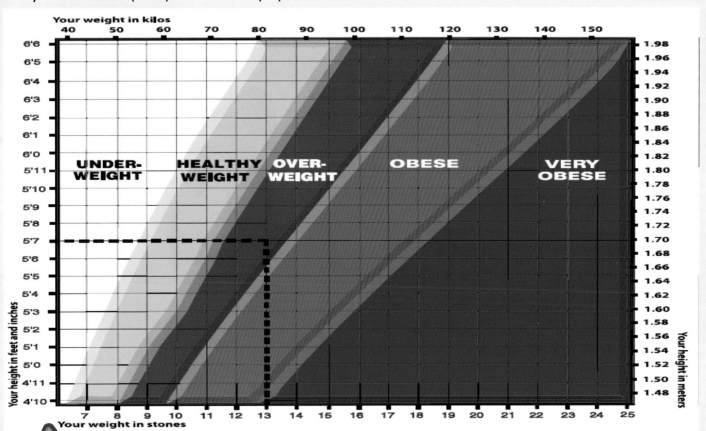

Note: The good news is that losing even a small amount of weight [between 5-10 kg] and keeping it off will help to keep blood glucose at normal levels.

White/ Black People	South Asian People
Body Mass Index [BMI]	
Underweight = less than 18.5 Kg/m^2	Underweight = less than 18.5 Kg/m^2
Healthy weight = 18.5 to 24.9 Kg/m^2	Healthy weight = 18.5 to 22.9 Kg/m^2
Overweight = 25 to 29.9 Kg/m^2	Overweight = 23 to 24.9 Kg/m^2
Obese = 30 to 39.9 Kg/m^2	Obese = 25 to 34.9 Kg/m^2
Very obese = more than 40 Kg/m^2	Very obese = more than 35 Kg/m^2

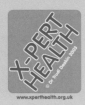

Waist Measurements

Waist measurements are now considered to be a more accurate measure of future health risk than body weight.

Knowing our waist measurement is more useful than simply knowing if you are a healthy weight, overweight or obese.

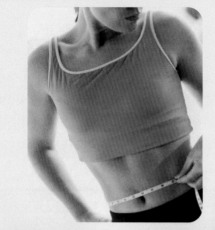

The location of your body fat makes a difference to your risk of diabetes and heart disease. People with excess fat around their waist (so-called "apple" shape) have a greater risk of dying from heart disease than people who carry weight on their hips and thighs (pear-shaped).

If you already have diabetes, carrying excess weight around the middle can make it more difficult to control.

People who have excess abdominal fat and who are in the overweight category, may not realise that they have a greater health risk than people in the obese category who are not carrying excess abdominal fat.

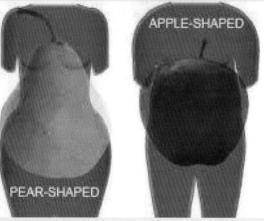

APPLE-SHAPED

PEAR-SHAPED

How to measure your waist and assess your health risk

1. Take the measurement without clothes to provide a more accurate measurement.

2. Place a tape evenly around the middle point of your waist by doing the following:

    a. find the top of your hip bone (you could mark it with a pen);
    b. find the very bottom of your rib-cage (you could mark it with a pen);
    c. the half-way point between the two marks is the correct position of your waist;
    d. place the tape evenly around this point to measure your waist size;
    e. write down this number in centimetres (cm) to the nearest mm.

3. Try to be relaxed and breathe out gently when reading the measurement.
   Do not 'suck in' the stomach.

4. Ensure the tape is snug but does not push tightly into the skin.

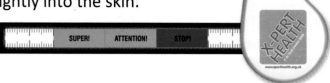

5. Take the measurement twice to check the reading.

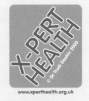

Waist Measurements

Please note: If you have difficulty feeling your rib-cage or hip bone or both, you may find it easier to place your hand, palm down, on your stomach. Place your middle finger on your tummy button and measure your waist just above your index finger.

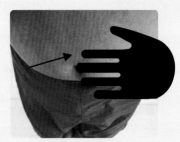

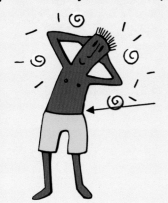

If you have a prolapse, which has resulted in your tummy button falling below your waist, you may find it easier to slightly bend to the side and measure your waist at the indent.

Consistency is the key! It is therefore advisable to measure your own waist circumference and use the same technique on each occasion.

What does my waist measurement mean?

Your waist should be under the measurements in the 'Healthy Waist' column below to protect your heart and to help you to look after your diabetes.

	Healthy Waist	Increased Risk	High Risk
For Men	Less than 94cm (about 37 inches)	More than or equal to 94cm (about 37 inches)	More than or equal to 102cm (about 40 inches)
For Women	Less than 80cm (about 32 inches)	More than or equal to 80cm (about 32 inches)	More than or equal to 88cm (about 35 inches)

You can record your waist measurement in the table below:

Today's Date	My Waist Measurement

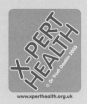

5 Essential Steps to Goal Setting

There is a lot of information, advice and instruction on adopting a healthy lifestyle. How many times have you been advised to do something such as give up smoking, lose weight, drink less alcohol? Have you always been able to make these changes when advised to do so?

You are the best person to decide what changes you want and are willing to make. People who come up with their own actions to address their concerns are much more successful in achieving them. We call this 'self-management' – as you are managing your own health. The X-PERT Diabetes Programme is designed not to tell you what to do but to provide you with the understanding and confidence so that you can make informed decisions regarding your lifestyle.

There are no rules for lifestyle options, just choices and consequences. Every week you will have the opportunity to work through the 5 steps to set goals and experiment with making lifestyle changes. Once your Health Profile has been completed with your own health results [on page 82/83 in the back of your handbook], ask yourself 'are you happy with your results or could you take steps to improve your health?' Put a cross (X) at the side of any of your health results that you would like to improve.

You might find it useful to complete 'Your Health Questions' on page 15 to identify a possible concern with your current health or lifestyle and reasons or motivation for change. Have a look at 'I want to.......' on page 16, which gives some pointers for improving your health results. Use the goal setting form on page 17 that has been shown to be very effective in helping you make long-term lifestyle changes. On page 18, you have the opportunity to think about things that will both *help you* and *stop you* reaching your goal. Increasing motivation for change and reducing the barriers may help you achieve your goals.

Step 1: What is my biggest concern about my health?

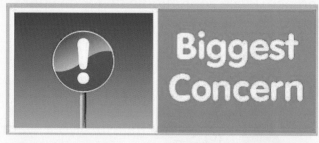

Step 2: How do I feel about the concern?

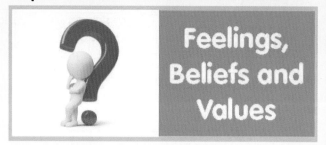

Step 3: What steps could I take to tackle the concern?

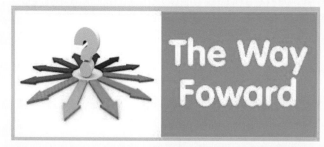

Step 4: What is the first step I'm going to take?

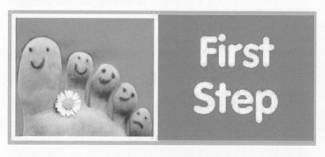

Step 5: What happened? Did it work?

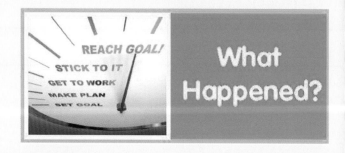

Your Health Questions

1) Do you feel healthy at the moment? _____

2) What would you have to do to improve your health? _____

3) Is there *one* thing that you can do to improve your health?

_____

4) What will you gain if you change? _____

5) What will be the most difficult thing about changing? _____

6) How will you cope with this? _____

7) What would be the worst thing that could happen if you don't change?

_____

8) What is one nice thing you could do for yourself after you make each lifestyle change?

_____

9) Have you any ideas about what will work? _____

10) What have you tried in the past? _____

11) Why do you think that did/didn't work? _____

12) What do you need to do to get started? _____

13) Does this sound like something you can do? _____

14) Are you sure this is something you want to do? _____

15) How confident are you that you can do it? _____

Scale 0 (not confident) to 10 (very confident)

If score is below 7 - explore why .... perhaps aim for smaller goal!

16) When would be a good time to start? _____

17) Make sure it is **S**pecific **M**easurable **A**ttainable **R**elevant **T**ime-Bound (SMART)

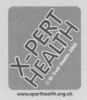

I Want To......

Lower my triglycerides

Is it possible to:
- lower your blood glucose levels?
- reduce sweet carbohydrate foods and drinks (including unsweetened fruit juice)
- reduce your alcohol intake?
- eat oily fish once or twice per week?
- cut back on calories?
- lose weight if overweight?
- increase physical activity?

Improve my blood glucose levels

Are you:
- eating too much carbohydrate?
- eating too much quick releasing carbohydrate?
- doing enough physical activity?
- overweight and need to lose weight?

Improve my bad "lethal" cholesterol [LDL]

Is it possible to:
- reduce the amount of saturated (animal) fat in your diet?
- choose foods high in soluble fibre such as oats and pulses?
- increase fruit and vegetables?
- use monounsaturated oils and spreads?
- have less processed foods?
- eat wholegrain bread, cereal and nuts
- lose weight if overweight
- increase physical activity

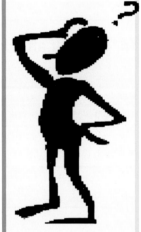

Lose weight

Try:
- burning more calories by doing more aerobic physical activity such as walking
- building lean body mass by resistance training such as water aerobics
- reducing calorie intake by having smaller portion sizes, reducing the fat content of the diet or cutting out snacks
- staving off hunger by having regular meals
- reducing temptation to snack between meals by having sufficient lean protein at mealtimes to keep you fuller for longer
- avoiding additional calories from alcohol

Lower my blood pressure

Try:
- reducing or omitting salt from cooking
- not adding salt to food at the table
- reducing processed foods
- increasing fruit and vegetables
- eating wholegrain bread, cereal and nuts
- eating sufficient low fat milk and dairy products
- attending smoking cessation sessions
- losing weight if overweight
- identifying coping strategies to deal with stress
- increasing physical activity
- taking blood pressure medication as prescribed

Increase my good "healthy" cholesterol [HDL]

Are you:
- achieving 30 minutes of physical activity five times a week?
- having between 5 and 9 portions of fruit and vegetables each day?
- using monounsaturated oils and spreads in preference to saturated and polyunsaturated fats?

N.B. Having a small amount of alcohol (equivalent to 1-2 units/day) may help to increase HDL cholesterol

Setting A Goal: My Health Results

1. What is my biggest concern about my health results?

_____

_____

2. How do I feel about the concern? What are my beliefs and values about this concern?

_____

_____

3. What steps could I take to tackle the concern?

_____

_____

4. What is the first step I'm going to take?

What? _____

When?_____

Why? _____

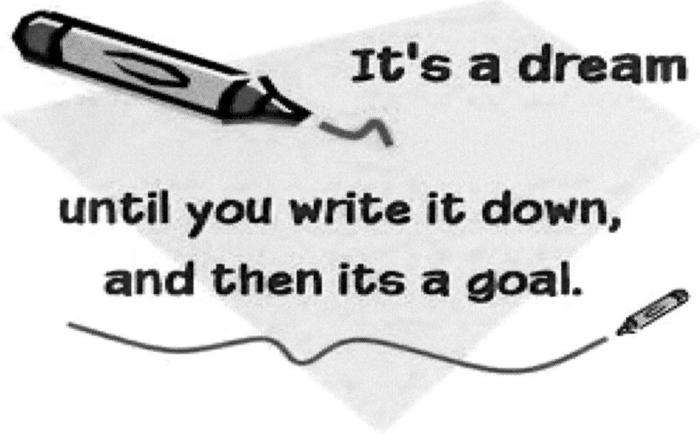

It's a dream until you write it down, and then its a goal.

5. What happened? Did it work? How do I know?

_____

_____

How confident am I that I can make the first step? (circle)

0   1   2   3   4   5   6   7   8   9   10

not at all certain   totally certain

If you score below 7 - explore why ..... perhaps aim for a smaller goal!

Tick each day you achieve your goal and note comments

Monday   _____

Tuesday   _____

Wednesday _____

Thursday   _____

Friday   _____

Saturday   _____

Sunday   _____

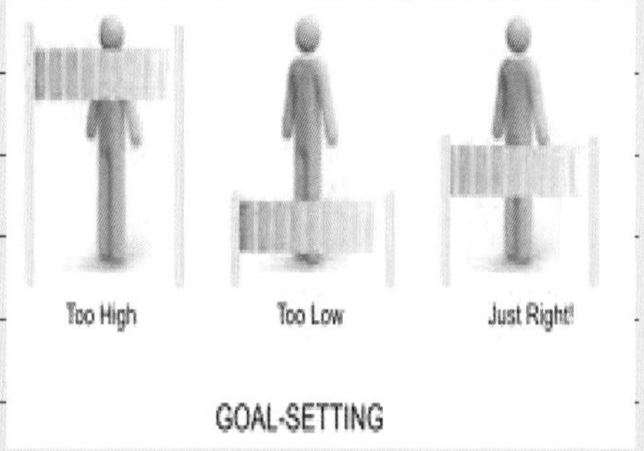

Too High   Too Low   Just Right!

GOAL-SETTING

Making changes to your lifestyle is not easy. When you are ready to make a change it can be helpful to plan how you will reach your goal. Thinking about the things in your life that are helpful and the things that are unhelpful will make it easier for you to plan changes.

Things that will STOP me reaching my goal

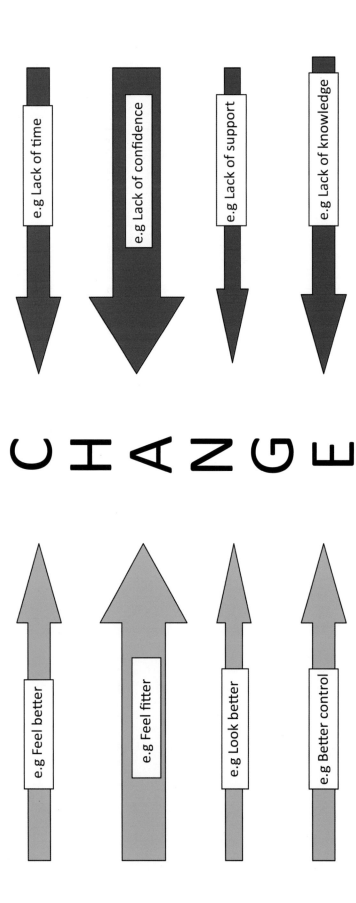

- e.g Lack of time
- e.g Lack of confidence
- e.g Lack of support
- e.g Lack of knowledge

C H A N G E

Things that will HELP me reach my goal

- e.g Feel better
- e.g Feel fitter
- e.g Look better
- e.g Better control

1) Can you add any things that will help you reach your goal?

2) Can you think of any ways to make one or more of the helpful things more important to you?

3) Can you remove any things that will stop you from reaching your goal?

4) Can you think of any ways to overcome the things that stop you reaching your goal?

18

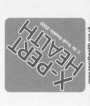

Section 2: Weight Management

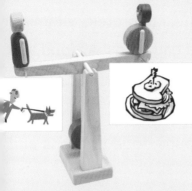

Balance food & activity

Energy Balance

We need nutrients to keep healthy. The three main nutrients in food (carbohydrate, fat and protein) provide us with energy (calories). In theory, energy balance is simple. If the calories you take in from food and drink are equal to the calories you burn through activity and carrying out body functions such as breathing, your weight will remain stable. To lose weight you need to take in fewer calories and/or burn more calories with activity. To gain weight you need to take in more calories and/or burn fewer during activity.

Main Message: On average, women require 2000 calories each day to maintain their weight and men require 2500 calories. But if you are small or inactive you will require fewer calories each day.

Remember: fat and alcohol contain the most calories!

1g fat contains 9 calories

1g alcohol contains 7 calories

1g carbohydrate contains 4 calories

1g protein contains 4 calories

Are crash diets the long-term solution to permanent weight loss?

- Going on a strict diet can appear to be successful initially but the weight loss is mainly short-term energy reserves and water.

- Weight loss slows down because losing fat is a much slower process than losing water.

- The body detects that food intake has been dramatically reduced and stops burning as many calories to guard against starvation.

- It's only a matter of time before the craving for high fat and sugary food starts and a struggle develops to fight those cravings.

- It is rare to resist such cravings for long and the 'diet' is usually broken.

- Sensible eating (instead of dieting), which allows people to continue to eat their favourite foods in small amounts and simultaneously increase their physical activity levels resulting in a deficit of 500 calories a day, has been shown to be a more successful and desirable approach to losing weight.

Please note: Recent reports have suggested that following a very low calorie diet i.e. 600 calories per day for 8 weeks may dramatically improve the way that the body copes with glucose allowing the diagnosis of diabetes to be reversed. Other reports have indicated that intermittent fasting known as the 5:2 diet is an effective method for successful weight loss. Whilst there may be merit in trying these approaches, the research data is somewhat limited. It is therefore important to discuss any plans to try these approaches with your GP or diabetes team beforehand.

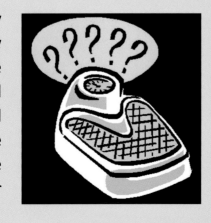

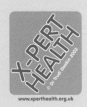

Eating for health and diabetes

Sensible eating provides us with all the 6 essentials for life: carbohydrate, fat, protein, vitamins, minerals and water. There is no need to separate foods into good and bad foods. All food and drink provide some of the essentials for life. It is important for health to learn about portion sizes and the recommended range of food portions from each food group.

The 'eatwell plate' is a model that helps us to understand food groups, food portions and healthy eating. The 5 food groups:

- **fruit & vegetables** provide a variety of vitamins and minerals, fibre and antioxidants and may help reduce the risk of heart disease, stroke and some cancers;

- **starchy carbohydrates** are a good source of energy and also provide us with fibre, calcium, iron and B vitamins;

- **protein foods** are essential for growth and repair of the body;

- **milk & dairy foods** provide us with calcium which is essential for healthy bones;

- **fatty and sugary foods** are not actually needed (essential fats are found in the other food groups) but eating in moderation can form part of a healthy diet.

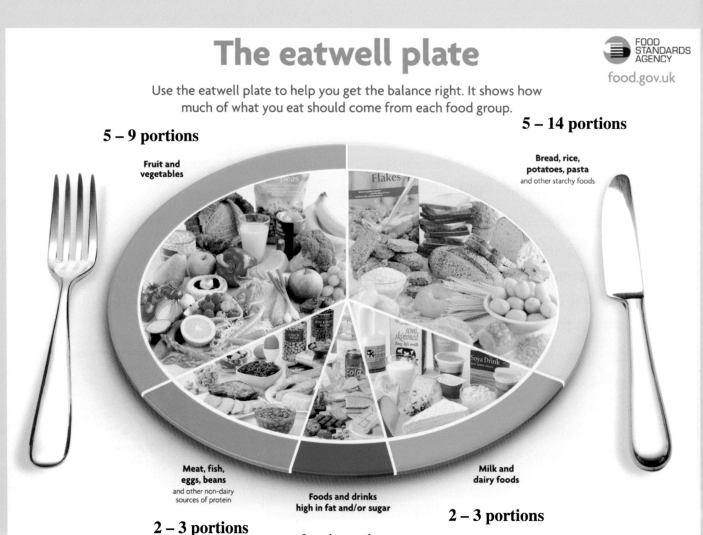

The eatwell plate

Use the eatwell plate to help you get the balance right. It shows how much of what you eat should come from each food group.

FOOD STANDARDS AGENCY
food.gov.uk

5 – 9 portions
Fruit and vegetables

5 – 14 portions
Bread, rice, potatoes, pasta and other starchy foods

Meat, fish, eggs, beans and other non-dairy sources of protein
2 – 3 portions

Foods and drinks high in fat and/or sugar
0 – 4 portions

Milk and dairy foods
2 – 3 portions

Eating for Health Guidance

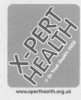

Key: tbs = tablespoon; tsp = teaspoon

Item		Food Group	Portion	Nutrition Information
Apple		Fruit & Vegetables	1 small 80g	Low calorie & fat free. Per 80g: 42 kcal, 9g carbs, 1g fibre
Apricots [Dried]		Fruit & Vegetables	6 pieces (30g)	Low fat, high fibre, slow-releasing. Per 30g: 72 kcal, 17g carbs, 2g fibre.
Aubergine		Fruit & Vegetables	1/3 (80g)	Low calorie & fat free. Per 80g: 13 kcal, 2g carbs, 2g fibre.
Avocado		Fruit & Vegetables	1/2 (80g)	Per 80g: 152 kcal, 16g fat, 3g saturates, 10g monounsatures, 2g carbs, 3g fibre.
Bacon, Unsmoked Rindless Back		Meat, Fish & Alternatives	4 rashers (85g cooked)	Per 85g grilled: 268 kcal, 22g fat, 7g saturates, 0g carbs, 3g salt [per rasher: 67 kcal, 6g fat & 2g saturates].
Baked Beans		Meat, Fish & Alternatives	1/2 large tin or small tin (~200g)	Per 200g: 164 kcal, 0g fat, 27g carbs, 8g fibre, 2g salt. Slow-release/soluble fibre.
Basmati Rice		Starchy Carbohydrates	2 tbs cooked (100g)	Low fat, moderate-releasing energy. 2 tbs cooked rice = approx 30g carbs.
Beefburger		Meat, Fish & Alternatives	1x small burger (85g)	Homemade burgers healthier if lean mince used. Onions/oatmeal can also be added.
Beef Steak Mince, Lean		Meat, Fish & Alternatives	85g (cooked) 120g (raw)	Per 85g (cooked): 155 kcal, 10g fat, 5g saturates, 0g carbs, 0g fibre, trace salt [extra lean mince fat = 5g/ 85g].
Biscuits, Oat e.g. Hobnobs		Fat & Sugary Foods	1	High in fat & sugar. Per biscuit: 73 kcal, 9g carbs, 3g fat & 0.3g saturates.
Breakfast Bar		Starchy Carbohydrates	1 small (25g)	Can be a good snack, need to read labels for fat & sugar content. Per Fitnesse Cereal Bar: 90 kcal, 18g carbs & 2g fat.
Broccoli		Fruit & Vegetables	3 tbs (80g)	Low calorie & fat free. Per 80g: 26 kcal, 1g carbs, 2g fibre.
Cauliflower		Fruit & Vegetables	3 tbs (80g)	Low calorie & fat free. Per 80g: 27 kcal, 2g carbs, 1g fibre.
Cereal: Just Right Fruit & Fibre		Starchy Carbohydrates	4 tbs (40g)	Low fat, high fibre cereal. 40g portion + 125ml semi-skimmed milk: 204 kcal, 37g carbs, 3g fat, 2g saturates & 2g fibre.
Chapatti Flour		Starchy Carbohydrates	1/2 chapatti (40g)	Half the weight of a chapatti is carbs: 1 x 80g chapatti (20cm across) = 40g carbs.
Cream Cheese		Milk & Dairy Foods	2 tsp (30g)	Per 30g: 75 kcal, 7g fat, 4g saturates, 1g carbs, 0.3g salt [Light = 4g fat, Extra light = 1g fat].
Cheese, Mature White Cheddar		Milk & Dairy Foods	Matchbox size (30g)	Per 30g: 125 kcal, 11g fat, 7g saturates. [Superlite 84 kcal, 5g fat, 0.4g saturates].
Cheese, Natural Cottage		Milk & Dairy Foods	2 tbs (80g)	Per 80g: 54 kcal, 0.1g fat & 2g carbs.

Eating for Health Guidance

Key: tbs = tablespoon; tsp = teaspoon

Item		Food Group	Portion	Nutrition Information
Chicken, Whole		Meat, Fish & Alternatives	85g cooked (120g raw)	Per 85g cooked (no skin): 136 kcal, 4g fat, 1g saturates, 0g carbs.
Chocolate, Dairy Milk		Fat & Sugary Foods	1 small bar (21g)	21g Bar = 110 Kcal, 6g fat, 4g saturates, 12g carbs, 0.1g fibre.
Chocolate, Dark (70% cocoa)		Fat & Sugary Foods	2 to 4 squares (20g)	Per 20g (1/5 100g bar): 115 kcal, 8g fat, 5g saturates, 7g carbs, 2g fibre.
Courgettes		Fruit & Vegetables	1/2 a large one (80g)	Low calorie & fat free. Per 80g: 14 kcal, 1g carbs, 0.7g fibre.
Cream, Whipped in can		Fat & Sugary Foods	1 tbs (12.5g)	Per 12.5g: 43 kcal, 4g fat, 3g saturates, 1g carbs.
Cucumber		Fruit & Vegetables	6 to 7cm (80g)	Low calorie & fat free. Per 80g: 8 kcal, 1g carbs, 0.5g fibre.
Dressing, Light Herb & Garlic		Fat & Sugary Foods	1 tbs (15ml)	Per 15ml: 17 kcal, 1g fat, 0.1g saturates, 2g carbs, 0g fibre, 0.3g salt.
Eggs		Meat, Fish & Alternatives	2 eggs (100g)	Per 2 eggs (100g): 151 kcal, 11g fat, 3g saturates, 4g monounsaturates, 0g carbs, 0.3g salt, 200mg cholesterol. Unlikely to increase blood cholesterol levels unless eaten to excess.
Fanta Orange		Fat & Sugary Foods	1 glass (250ml)	Per glass (250ml): 75 kcal, 0g fat, 18g carbs, 0g fibre. Per bottle (500ml): 150 kcal, 0g fat, 36g carbs, 0g fibre.
Fish, Oily [smoked mackerel]		Meat, Fish & Alternatives	100g (cooked)	Per 100g: 293 kcal, 24g fat, 5g saturates, 2g salt, 4.5g omega-3 fatty acids [good source that reduce triglycerides].
Flour Tortillas		Starchy Carbohydrates	1 (40g)	Per serving (40g): 140 kcal, 5g fat, 2g saturates, 20g carbs, 2g fibre, 1g salt.
Fruit Cocktail in Juice		Fruit & Vegetables	3 tbs (80g)	Per serving (80g): 40 kcal, 0g fat, 10g carbs, 1g fibre, 0g salt. Fewer carbs when tinned in juice rather than syrup.
Garden Peas, Fresh/Frozen		Fruit & Vegetables	3 tbs (80g)	Per serving (80g): 54 kcal, 1g fat, 6g carbs, 5g fibre, 0g salt. Good source of soluble fibre.
Gram Flour for Chapatti		Starchy Carbohydrates	25g flour [1/2 small chapatti]	Per 50g serving (1 sm chapatti): 180 kcal, 3g fat, 30g carbs, 5g fibre, 0g salt. Concentrated carbohydrate source.

Eating for Health Guidance

Key: tbs = tablespoon; tsp = teaspoon

Item		Food Group	Portion	Nutrition Information
Granulated Sugar, Half Spoon		Fat & Sugary Foods	1/2 tsp (2g)	Per 1/2 tsp (2g): 8 kcal, 0g fat, 2g carbs. 1/2 tsp = 1 tsp normal sugar because sweeter [Sugar = 20 kcal, 0g fat, 5g carbs].
Ham, Baked		Meat, Fish & Alternatives	3 slices (85g)	Per 85g: 102 kcal, 3g fat, 1g saturates, 1g carbs, 0g fibre, 1.7g salt. Red meat is a good source of iron.
Jam		Fat & Sugary Foods	1 heaped tsp (15g)	Per serving (15g): 40 kcal, 0g fat, 10g carbs, 0.2g fibre [reduced sugar jam contains slightly less carbs: 6g per serving].
Lettuce		Fruit & Vegetables	1 small bowl (80g)	Low calorie & fat free. Per 80g: 18 kcal, 3g carbs, 2g fibre.
Mayonnaise		Fat & Sugary Foods	2 tsp (10g)	High fat. Per serving (10g): 72 kcal, 8g fat, 1g saturated fat, 1g omega-3, 0.2g salt.
Meringue Nests		Fat & Sugary Foods	1 (13g)	Per nest (13g): 52 kcal, 0g fat, 12g carbs, 0g fibre, 0g salt.
Milk, skimmed or semi-skimmed		Milk & Dairy Foods	1 medium glass (200ml)	Low in fat, good source of calcium. Per 200ml: 98 kcal, 3g fat, 2g saturates, 10g carbs, 0g fibre, 0.3g salt.
Mushrooms		Fruit & Vegetables	3 tbs (80g)	Low calorie & fat free. Per 80g: 10 kcal, 0.3g carbs, 1g fibre.
Naan Bread		Starchy Carbohydrates	1/2 naan (50g)	Per naan (100g): 300 kcal, 12g fat, 2g saturates, 41g carbs, 2g fibre, 0.8g salt.
Oat Crisp/ Krunchies		Starchy Carbohydrates	3-4 tbs (30g)	Per 30g serving: 109 kcal, 2g fat, 0.4g saturates, 18g carbs, 4g fibre [1g soluble], 0.2g salt. Good source of soluble fibre.
Oats, Porridge		Starchy Carbohydrates	27g sachet (2 tbs)	Per 27g serving: 98 kcal, 2g fat, 0.4g saturates, 16g carbs, 3g fibre (1g soluble), 0g salt. Slow-release energy.
Oil, Pure Vegetable (100% rapeseed in the UK)		Fat & Sugary Foods	1 dessert spoon (10ml)	Per 10ml: 83 kcal, 9g fat, 0.6g saturates, 5g monounsaturates, 3g polyunsaturates. No carbs, fibre or salt. High fat but low saturated fat.
Orange		Fruit & Vegetables	1 small 80g edible portion	Low calorie & fat free. Per 80g: 30 kcal, 7g carbs, 1.4g fibre.
Orange Juice,100% Pure Squeezed		Fruit & Vegetables	Small glass (150ml)	Per 150ml: 68 kcal, 0.2g fat, 0g saturates, 15g carbs, 0.2g fibre, 0g salt. Can only count as 1 portion of fruit or vegetables.
Peas, Mushy (Tinned)		Fruit & Vegetables	2 tbs (80g)	Per 80g: 66 kcal, 0.4g fat, 0.2g saturates, 11g carbs, 2g fibre, 0.5g salt. Good source of soluble fibre.

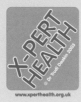

Eating for Health Guidance

Key: tbs = tablespoon; tsp = teaspoon

Item		Food Group	Portion	Nutrition Information
Pineapple		Fruit & Vegetables	2 thin slices (80g)	Low calorie & fat free. Per 80g: 42 kcal, 10g carbs, 1g fibre.
Pizza		Starchy Carbs (base) + Milk & Dairy (cheese)	1/4 12" deep pan (175g)	High fat/carb. Per 1/4: 500 kcal, 19g fat, 9g saturates, 55g carbs, 2g fibre, 2.2g salt [1/4 thin crust pizza: 189 kcal, 8g fat, 5g saturates, 20g carbs].
Poppadums		Fat & Sugary Foods	2 (22g)	Per 2: 110 kcal, 5g fat, 0.4g saturates, 9g carbs, 2g fibre, 0.8g salt.
Pork Leg Steaks		Meat, Fish & Alternatives	85g (cooked) 120g (raw)	Per 85g (grilled and fat trimmed off): 179 kcal, 7g fat, 3g saturates, 0g carbs, 0.3g salt. Good source of iron.
Pork Pie		Fat & Sugary Foods	1/2 individual (70g)	High in total and saturated fat. Per 70g: 263 kcal, 19g fat, 7g saturates, 15g carbs, 1.5g fibre, 1g salt.
Potatoes		Starchy Carbohydrates	3 small new/ 1 medium old (100g)	Fat free. Old potatoes = quick-releasing energy. New potatoes = moderate-releasing. Per 100g: 78 kcal, 0g fat, 17g carbs, 1g fibre, 0g salt.
Prawns, Cooked & Peeled		Meat, Fish & Alternatives	4 tbs cooked (140g)	Per 140g: 91 kcal, 1g fat, 0.4g saturates, 0g carbs/fibre, 1.8g salt. Almost fat free. Watch the fat content in the sauce!
Pulses for Dhal		Meat, Fish & Alternatives	3 - 4tbs cooked [~ 100g]	Per 100g (cooked): 99 kcal, 1g fat, 0g saturates, 20g carbs, 5g fibre, 0g salt. Good source of soluble fibre.
Red Lentils		Meat, Fish & Alternatives	3 - 4tbs cooked [~ 100g]	Per 100g (cooked): 101 kcal, 0.4g fat, 0g saturates, 18g carbs, 3g fibre, 0g salt. Good source of soluble fibre.
Salmon Fillets		Meat, Fish & Alternatives	100g (cooked)	Per 100g (grilled): 237 kcal, 14g fat, 3g saturates, 0g carbs, 0.6g fibre, 0.2g salt, 3g omega-3 (reduce triglycerides).
Sardines in Tomato Sauce		Meat, Fish & Alternatives	100g (cooked)	Per 100g: 182 kcal, 13g fat, 2g saturates, 0g carbs, 0.4g fibre, 0.8g salt, 4g omega-3 (reduce triglycerides).
Seeded Batch		Starchy Carbohydrates	1 slice (45.6g)	Per slice: 137 kcal, 4g fat, 1g saturates, 18g carbs, 3g fibre, 0.5g salt. Moderate-release energy.
Shredded Wheat with Berries		Starchy Carbohydrates	4 tbs (40g)	Low fat, high fibre. Per 40g: 139 kcal, 0.6g fat, 0g saturates, 15g carbs, 3g fibre, 0g salt.
Spaghetti		Starchy Carbohydrates	25g raw/ 2 tbs (50g) cooked	Per 50g (cooked): 78 kcal, 0.3g fat, 0g saturates, 16g carbs, 1g fibre, 0g salt. Slow-release energy.
Spread, Olive Oil		Fat & Sugary Foods	2tsp (14g)	Good source of monounsaturated fat. Per 14g: 75 kcal, 8g fat, 2g saturates, 4g monounsaturates, 0g carbs, 0.2g salt.

Eating for Health Guidance

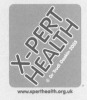

Key: tbs = tablespoon; tsp = teaspoon

Item		Food Group	Portion	Nutrition Information
Splenda Sweetener		Fat & Sugary Foods	2 tsp (10g)	Per 10g: 4 kcal, 0g fat, 10g carbs, 0g fibre, 0g salt. Half the calories & carbs of sugar.
Tomato		Fruit & Vegetables	1 medium or 8 cherry (80g)	Per 80g: 15 kcal, 0g fat, 3g carbs, 1g fibre, 0g salt. Cooked tomatoes are a good source of lycopene.
Trout, Whole		Meat, Fish & Alternatives	100g fillet	Per 100g (grilled): 173 kcal, 9g fat, 4g saturates, 0g carbs, 0g fibre, 0.2g salt, 1g omega-3 (reduce triglycerides).
Tuna Chunks in Spring Water		Meat, Fish & Alternatives	2/3 tin [100g drained]	Per 100g: 100 kcal, 0.6g fat, 0.8g salt. [Fresh tuna = more omega 3. Tinned in brine = more salt, in oil = more fat].
Utterly Butterly		Fat & Sugary Foods	2 tsp (14g)	Good source: monounsaturates. Per 14g: 63 kcal, 7g fat, 2g saturates, 3g mono-unsaturates. [Utterly Butterly v Butter = 49% v 80% fat, 13% v 54% saturates]
Weetabix/Oatibix		Starchy Carbohydrates	1 biscuit or 1-2 tbs bites (20g)	High fibre, low fat. Moderate-release energy. Per 20g: 80 kcal, 2g fat, 0g saturates, 14g carbs, 2g fibre, 0g salt.
Yoghurt, Muller Light		Milk & Dairy Foods	1 pot (175g)	Per 175g: 89 kcal, 0.2g fat, 14g carbs, 26% of daily calcium requirement.
Yoghurt, Shape		Milk & Dairy Foods	1 pot (120g)	Per 120g: 79 kcal, 0.1g fat, 13g carbs, 26% of daily calcium requirement.

Please note: portion sizes and discussion points may vary due to different ingredients used by manufacturers. New products that become available may differ in nutritional content.

Hints for Weight Loss

Weight loss occurs when there are more calories being used up for energy than there are entering the body through food and drink. Therefore to lose weight you need to eat less, be more active or a combination of the two.

Dietary options to reduce calories

1. Cut down on the amount of food eaten e.g. reduce portion sizes.
2. Reduce fat content of the diet (fat contains more than twice the calories than carbohydrate or protein) [see low v high fat diet on page 26].
3. Slightly increase protein content whilst reducing carbohydrate as this may increase the feeling of fullness and reduce snacking between meals.

Research has shown that a combination of reducing calories and increasing activity is the most effective way to achieve long-term weight loss targets. We call this an energy deficit. A daily energy deficit of 500 calories over a week will result in 0.5kg [1lb] weight loss and over a month, 2.5kg [5lb] weight loss. Examples of 500 calorie energy deficits can be seen on page 27.

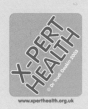

Comparison of Low Fat and High Fat Diet

Please note: Kcal = calories, Carbs = carbohydrate

Low Fat Diet	Kcal	Fat (g)	Carbs (g)	High Fat Diet	Kcal	Fat (g)	Carbs (g)
Breakfast				**Breakfast**			
Fruit & Fibre (4 tbsp/30g)	140	2.0	28	Porridge oats* (30g)	110	2.4	18.6
Semi-skimmed milk (125 ml)	60	2.0	6	Full fat milk (200ml)	130	8.0	9.4
Granary bread (1 slice/40g)	95	0.8	18	Toast (1 slice/40g)	102	1.0	19.5
Jam (1 tsp/15g)	40	-	10	Margarine (2 tsp/14g)	96	9.4	0.2
Pure orange juice (200 ml)	86	-	18	Pure orange juice (200 ml)	86	-	18
Snack				**Snack**			
Piece of fruit (80g)	46	-	18	Chocolate digestive (x2)	165	8.2	21
Lunch				**Lunch**			
Carrot/butterbean soup ½ tin	117	4.0	17	Grilled sausages (x3)	474	33.6	23
Pitta bread (x1)	190	1.0	38	Bread (x2 slices/80g)	204	2.0	39
Salad (tomato/lettuce)	20	-	4	Margarine (4 tsp/28g)	192	18.8	0.4
Salmon (tinned, 50g)	75	4.0	-	Yoghurt (full fat 200g)	224	7.2	33
Reduced fat mayo (1 tsp/5g)	30	3.0	0.7				
Low fat yoghurt (200g pot)	106	0.2	17				
Snack				**Snack**			
Reduced fat crisps (1 pk/30g)	132	5.9	16	Packet of crisps (30g)	183	11.4	17.3
Evening Meal				**Evening Meal**			
Pork loin (100g)	129	2.2	-	Chicken & Leek Pie (1 individual)	555	33.8	41
4 x new potato (200g)	152	0.2	37	Chips (200g)	506	21.8	75
Carrots (2 tbsp /50g)	9	-	2.1	Peas (2 tbsp/80g)	60	0.8	8.4
Broccoli (3 tbsp /100g)	18	-	1.6	Apple Pie (1 individual)	500	25.2	62
Bisto (50 ml)	14	0.5	2.1	Single cream (80 ml)	158	15.2	3.1
Banana (100g)	79	0.3	19				
Low fat ice-cream (1 scoop)	80	1.5	15				
Supper				**Supper**			
Options drink	40	1.3	5.5	Cream crackers (x2)	66	2.4	10.0
Chocolate (4 squares/20g)	115	8.0	9.1	Cheddar cheese (50g)	205	17.2	-
				Margarine (2 tsp/14g)	96	9.4	0.2
				300ml lager / beer / cider	200	-	14.0
Milk in Drinks				**Milk in Drinks**			
Semi-skimmed milk (200ml)	98	3.4	10	Full fat milk (200ml)	132	8.0	9.6
TOTAL (g) Percentage (%)	**1871 Kcal**	**40g 19%**	**292g 62%**	**TOTAL Percentage (%)**	**4420 Kcal**	**234g 48%**	**423g 38%**

Please Note: This information was correct at the time of printing but different brands may have a different nutritional content.

*Porridge oats are not high fat but making porridge using full fat milk adds unnecessary fat and calories.

www.xperthealth.org.uk

500 Kcal Energy Deficit

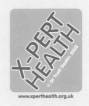

Research has shown that a combination of reducing calories and increasing activity is the most effective way to achieve long-term weight loss targets. We call this an energy deficit. A daily energy deficit of 500 calories will result in 0.5Kg (1lb) fat loss in 1 week and 2.5Kg (5lb) fat loss in 1 month. This can be achieved by increasing physical activity [burning additional calories] and eating less [saving calories]. The examples below provide ideas about how to achieve a daily 500 calorie deficit. It is these small steps that can make all the difference!

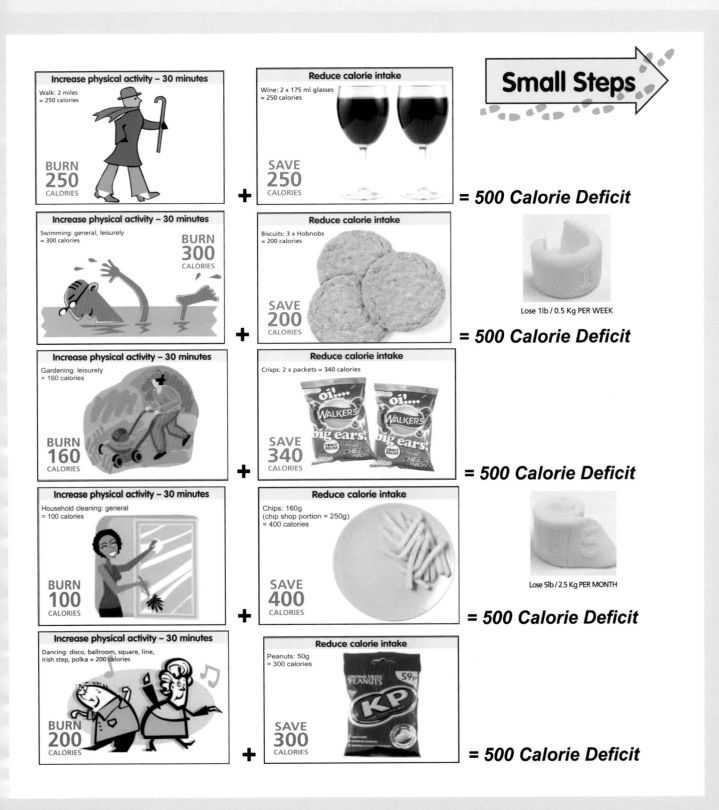

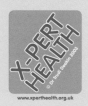

BENEFITS OF PHYSICAL ACTIVITY

General

* More energy

* Improved sleep at night

* Increased strength/greater stamina

* Lower risk of heart disease & stroke

* Reduces depression

* Healthier bones

* Helps weight control

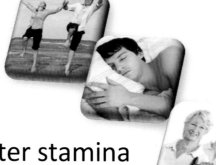

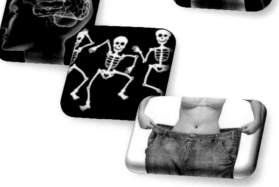

Benefits for Diabetes

* Improves blood glucose control (HbA1c)

* Reduces heart disease/stroke risk by 35-50%

* Improves blood cholesterol levels

* Reduces blood pressure

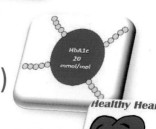

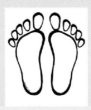

Every Step Counts

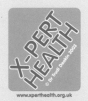

Guidance: 30 to 60 minutes moderate-intensity or 15 minutes vigorous-intensity physical activity at least 5 times per week - build up in bouts of 10 minutes - small changes make the difference

Did you know? When being physically active, you do not need insulin to unlock the door into the body cell. The glucose can enter on its own! Physical activity really helps to control blood glucose.

Two types of physical activity can improve health and diabetes control:

1. **Aerobic "cardiovascular"** activities train the heart to become fitter, reduce blood pressure and also burn calories. Examples are walking, jogging, swimming, dancing and cycling.

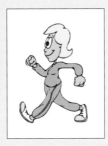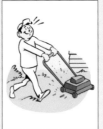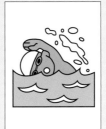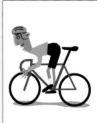

2. **Resistance training** is any exercise that will give resistance against your muscles such as weight lifting or using special training elastic bands. This helps to build lean body mass (muscle) that keeps the body supple. Muscle also burns more calories than fat.

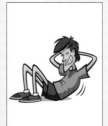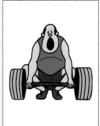

A STEPOMETER or PEDOMETER is a handy way to measure your aerobic activity levels throughout the day. Stepometers and pedometers can be purchased in sports shops and pharmacies.

- ○ Simply press the button and start walking..... the STEPOMETER will count every step you take or the PEDOMETER will measure the distance you walk.
- ○ Clip it onto your belt or waist band and off you go!
- ○ At the start of each day, reset the STEPOMETER/PEDOMETER by pressing the button.
- ○ Start off slowly. See how much activity you have achieved by checking your STEPOMETER/ PEDOMETER at the end of each day.
- ○ Day by day, add a little more activity to your day and remember - Every Step Counts!
- ○ For optimum health, experts recommend that we aim for around 10,000 steps every day [10,000 steps is equal to approximately 5 miles].
- ○ Don't be put off if you start at 1,000 or 2,000 steps [$^1/_2$-1 mile]. Each day, do a few more steps aiming for a target of 10,000 (5 miles) - Every Step Counts!

Your STEPOMETER/PEDOMETER counts every step, including your everyday chores like vacuuming; walking to the shops; walking from the bedroom to the bathroom; so every step you take will get you closer to the recommended 10,000 steps (5 miles) per day.

Tips For Building Those Steps
- ○ Walk to work or to the shops
- ○ Take the stairs instead of the lift
- ○ Log your progress by keeping an activity diary
- ○ Get off the bus a stop or two earlier
- ○ Wear your STEPOMETER while doing household chores

REGULAR ACTIVITY + HEALTHY EATING = A HEALTHY WEIGHT

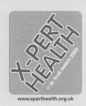

Eating Well for Diabetes

The Basis of Healthy Eating

Remember that all starchy carbohydrates digest in the gut and break down to glucose. Therefore be careful that you don't eat carbohydrates to excess.

- Oats and pulses are high in soluble fibre
- Try and include some wholegrain on a daily basis in breakfast cereals or bread
- New and sweet potatoes break down more slowly than old potatoes
- Pasta is a slow releasing carb but watch the portion size and avoid creamy sauces
- Basmati rice releases glucose into the blood more slowly than long-grain rice

Try to have a variety of fruit and vegetables every day.

- Fresh, frozen, stewed fruits
- Berries
- Grapes & slices of tropical fruit
- Tinned fruit in juice
- Unsweetened fruit juice or dried fruit
- Fresh, frozen & tinned vegetables
- Salad vegetables

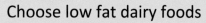

Spread your fruit throughout the day to avoid a large carbohydrate load.

Choose low fat dairy foods

- Low fat or fat free milk
- Diet or very low fat yoghurt/fromage frais
- Low fat or cottage cheese
- Low fat milk puddings

Try lean protein foods

- Lean red meat/poultry without the skin
- White fish e.g. cod, haddock, whiting, plaice
- Peas, beans, lentils, nuts and seeds
- Oily fish

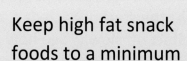

Keep high fat snack foods to a minimum
- Crisps, cakes, biscuits, chocolate, sweets, pies and puddings

Choose foods rich in monounsaturated fat and omega-3 fatty acids

- Olive oil or rapeseed oil (use sparingly)
- Olive oil/rapeseed spread e.g. Bertolli/Golden Olive/Utterly Butterly (use sparingly)
- Oily fish e.g. mackerel, salmon, sardines, trout, herring, pilchards, kippers.

Tips for Meals

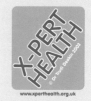

What can I choose for breakfast?

- For an energy boost have starchy carbohydrate at breakfast e.g. oat-based or wholegrain cereal or bread.

- Add low fat dairy foods to provide calcium e.g. low fat: milk, yoghurt or fromage frais.

- Add some fruit to increase fibre, vitamins and minerals e.g. fresh, tinned in natural juice or dried.

- A cooked breakfast for a change?
  Try a poached egg, baked beans, grilled tomato & mushrooms or increase your intake of omega-3 by having kippers.

What can I choose for my dinner?
Include a little starchy food
Be carbohydrate aware: make sure that your carb portions match your activity levels.

- Potatoes [boiled, mashed or roasted], pasta, noodles, rice, couscous, bulgar wheat........
- Add beans and lentils to stews and casseroles
- Use oats or oat bran to coat fish or chicken.
- Fill up by adding plenty of salad and/or vegetables [raw, steamed, boiled, stir-fried or roasted].
- For protein: include lean meat, poultry, oily fish, white fish, eggs or vegetarian sources such as Quorn, tofu, soya, peas, beans, lentils, seeds or nuts.

What foods can I choose for my lunch or tea?
Have one starchy food......
- Bread: all types but try to have wholegrain, granary, or any containing nuts, seeds, fruit
- Add lentils, beans, pasta shapes, peas, noodles or basmati rice to soups
- For a change try pasta or rice salads.

Add some protein........
- Slices of lean roast beef, pork, chicken or turkey to sandwiches or add to salads; grate low fat cheese & carrot together; use cottage cheese with dried apricots; try oily fish on toast - this can make paté when mixed with cottage cheese & lemon
- Try vegetarian protein sources such as Quorn, tofu, soya, pulses, seeds, nuts.

Have lots of vegetables and salad to provide colour, vitamins and to fill you up!

Snacks, desserts & supper

Keep to a minimum if trying to lose weight as snacks and desserts may add unnecessary carbs & calories. Carbohydrate load may be reduced by decreasing starchy carb intake in the savoury part of the meal.

- Fruit - fresh, tinned in natural juice (plain or with low fat yoghurt)
- Handful of dried fruit or unsalted nuts
- Low fat yoghurt or fromage frais
- Glass of low fat flavoured milk
- Small portion of cereal with low fat milk or handful of cereal e.g. Raisin Shreddies
- Fruit & Oat Ryvita
- Fruit scone or homemade fruit loaf
- Low fat milk pudding or oaty fruit crumble with low fat custard
- Meringue, fromage frais & fruit
- Stewed fruit and ice cream.
- Homemade cakes using healthy eating recipes

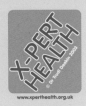

Setting a Goal:
Dietary Self-Assessment

Assess your diet to see how healthy it is

You can compare your daily intake of food to the healthy eating recommendations using the *eatwell plate* model. It is simple to do and provides you with immediate feedback about how healthy your diet is. To complete the dietary self-assessment follow these steps:

1. Think of your meals and snacks on a typical day (or yesterday). You may find it helpful to complete the blank Food Diary on page 33 to help you do this.

2. Complete the blank eatwell plate titled "what are you having?" on page 34 and for each food you have eaten, ask yourself: "where does this belong in the *eatwell plate*?" and "how many portions does this contain?"

3. Refer to 'What is a portion?' on page 36 or 'Eating for Health Guidance' (pages 21-25) to work out your portion sizes.

4. When you have finished completing the 'What are you having? eatwell plate' template with a typical day, add up the number of portions from each food group.

5. OPTIONAL: You can estimate total energy (calorie) intake by adding-up the number of calories consumed from each food group. To estimate calories, the following assumptions have been made:

   ○ 1 portion (P) of **fruit/vegetables** is 50 Kcal;
   ○ 1 portion (P) of starchy carbohydrate is 80 Kcal;
   ○ 1 portion (P) of milk & dairy is 100 Kcal;
   ○ 1 portion (P) of **protein foods** is 150 Kcal;
   ○ 1 portion (P) of **fatty/sugary foods** is 100 Kcal
   ○ 1 portion (P) of alcohol is 100 Kcal

   Have a look at the example of a 2130 Kcal eating plan' (page 35).

6. Count up the number of food portions in each section of the eatwell plate and complete the worksheet on page 37 'My Plan for Change' comparing your diet to the healthy eating recommendations and identifying goals for change.

7. Complete the goal setting form on page 38 to focus on a SMART goal to address your diet or activity levels over the following week.

Questions to ask yourself about your daily diet
- Am I eating between 5 and 9 portions of fruit & vegetables? Am I having enough variety?
- Am I eating the *right amount* of starchy carbohydrates to meet my activity levels (between 5 and 14 portions)? Am I having enough fibre?
- Am I having 2 to 3 portions of milk and dairy food? Am I choosing the low fat options?
- Am I having **2 to 3 portions of protein foods**? Am I choosing a variety of white/oily fish, lean meat, and vegetarian options such as pulses, nuts and seeds?
- Am I having **small quantities of fat and sugars** (between 0 and 4 portions)? Am I choosing monounsaturated oils and spreads?
- How many units of alcohol am I having? Am I sticking to 2 units (female) or 3 units (male)?

Food Diary

You may find it helpful to write down everything you eat and drink for one day. You can then use this information to compare how your own diet matches up to the advice on the eatwell plate.

Meal	Food or Drink & Description	How much (portion size)
Breakfast		
Lunch		
Evening Meal		
Snacks: (morning, afternoon and evening) if consumed in addition to meals		
Supper:		

N.B. If you found it helpful to keep a food diary you might like to use a note book to continue in the future.

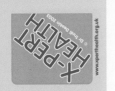

The 'eatwell plate' – What Are You Having?

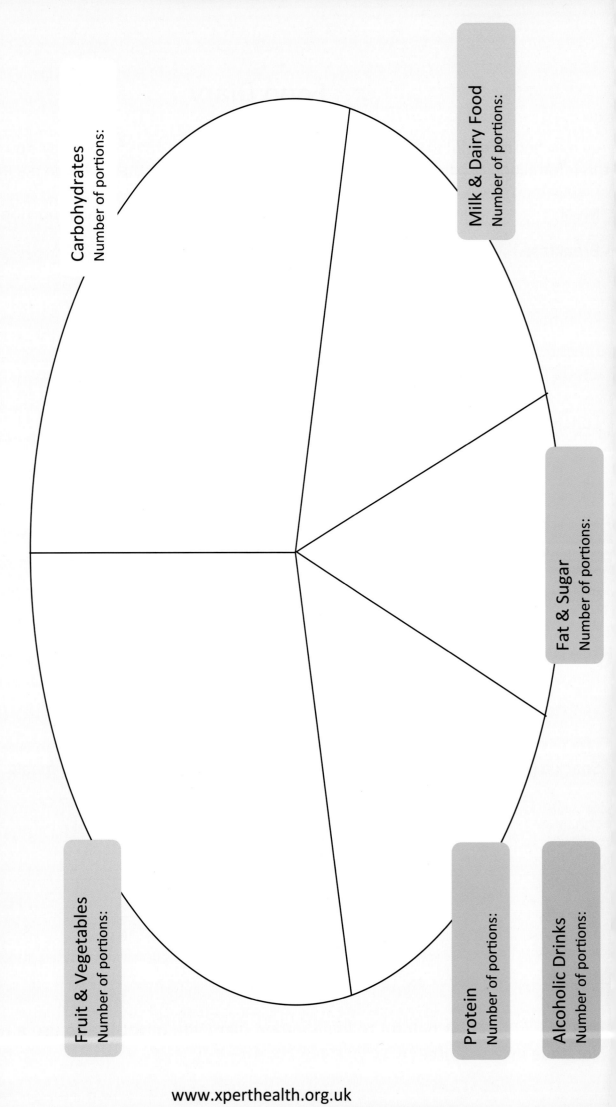

Carbohydrates
Number of portions:

Milk & Dairy Food
Number of portions:

Fat & Sugar
Number of portions:

Fruit & Vegetables
Number of portions:

Protein
Number of portions:

Alcoholic Drinks
Number of portions:

www.xperthealth.org.uk

Dietary Self-Assessment Example

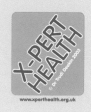

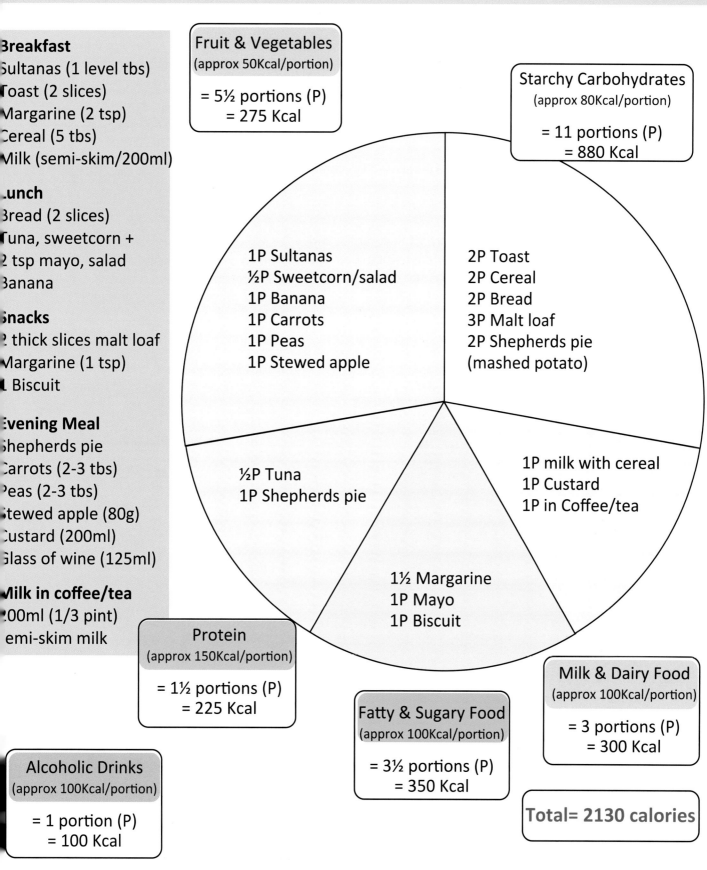

Breakfast
Sultanas (1 level tbs)
Toast (2 slices)
Margarine (2 tsp)
Cereal (5 tbs)
Milk (semi-skim/200ml)

Lunch
Bread (2 slices)
Tuna, sweetcorn +
2 tsp mayo, salad
Banana

Snacks
2 thick slices malt loaf
Margarine (1 tsp)
1 Biscuit

Evening Meal
Shepherds pie
Carrots (2-3 tbs)
Peas (2-3 tbs)
Stewed apple (80g)
Custard (200ml)
Glass of wine (125ml)

Milk in coffee/tea
200ml (1/3 pint)
semi-skim milk

Fruit & Vegetables
(approx 50Kcal/portion)

= 5½ portions (P)
= 275 Kcal

Starchy Carbohydrates
(approx 80Kcal/portion)

= 11 portions (P)
= 880 Kcal

1P Sultanas
½P Sweetcorn/salad
1P Banana
1P Carrots
1P Peas
1P Stewed apple

2P Toast
2P Cereal
2P Bread
3P Malt loaf
2P Shepherds pie
(mashed potato)

½P Tuna
1P Shepherds pie

1P milk with cereal
1P Custard
1P in Coffee/tea

1½ Margarine
1P Mayo
1P Biscuit

Protein
(approx 150Kcal/portion)

= 1½ portions (P)
= 225 Kcal

Fatty & Sugary Food
(approx 100Kcal/portion)

= 3½ portions (P)
= 350 Kcal

Milk & Dairy Food
(approx 100Kcal/portion)

= 3 portions (P)
= 300 Kcal

Total= 2130 calories

Alcoholic Drinks
(approx 100Kcal/portion)

= 1 portion (P)
= 100 Kcal

KEY: tbs = tablespoon   tsp = teaspoon   P = portion

What is a Portion?

FOOD GROUP	DAILY PORTIONS	WHAT IS A PORTION?
Bread, Cereals and Potato, Rice & Pasta (contains starchy carbohydrates)	**5 to 14 portions** [Note: most people will eat more than one portion of starchy carbohydrate at a meal as 1 serving often provides more than 1 portion of carbs e.g. 2 slices of bread = 2 portions; bowl of cereal = 2 or 3 portions, 1 baked potato = 3 portions, 200g pasta = 4 portions].	○ 2-4 tbs breakfast cereal (20-40g) ○ Slice of bread/toast (40g) ○ ½ teacake (40g) ○ ½ small pitta bread/chapatti (40g) ○ 1 to 2 tbsp (40-50g) rice/pasta ○ 2 crackers/4-6 chips (40-50g) ○ 2 new/baked/1-2 tbsp mashed potato(100-120g) ○ ½ scone/½ slice malt loaf (25g)
Fruit & Vegetables (contains fibre, vitamins and minerals)	**5 to 9 portions** Include a mixture of vegetables and fruit daily - at least 400g per day [Fresh, frozen, tinned or dried].	○ 2-3 tbsp vegetables (80g) ○ Side salad ○ Piece of fresh fruit (80g) ○ 3 tbsp stewed/tinned fruit (80g) ○ Small glass (150ml) fruit juice ○ Small cup grapes/cherries (80g) ○ 1 tbs dried fruit/3 dates or prunes
Meat, Fish, Poultry & Alternatives (contains protein)	**2 to 3 portions** Choose lower fat types [Note: a 3oz [85g] meat portion is the size of a deck of cards]	○ 3oz (85g) red meat, chicken or oily fish ○ 4-5 oz (120-140g) white fish (unbattered) ○ 2 eggs ○ ½ large tin or small tin (~200g) ○ 4 tbsp dish based on pulses/lentils/dhal ○ 2 tbsp nuts/peanut butter
Milk & Dairy Food (contains calcium)	**2 to 3 portions** Choose lower fat types [Note: a 1oz [30g] chunk of cheese is the size of a small matchbox]	○ ⅓ pint (200ml) milk ○ Small pot yoghurt/fromage frais ○ 2 tbsp cottage cheese ○ 1oz (30g) cheese ○ Small portion of custard (150ml)
Fatty & Sugary Foods	**0 to 4 portions** Remember the <u>type</u> of fat is important - choose monounsaturated fat where possible.	○ 2 tsp (14g) margarine/10ml oil ○ 2 tsp mayonnaise/salad dressing-10g ○ ½ sausage/rasher streaky bacon ○ 1 scoop ice cream (50g)/1 tbsp cream ○ 1 mini chocolate bar (21g)/choc biscuit ○ 2 - 3 boiled sweets/ ½ packet of crisps ○ 2 tsp sugar/jam/honey (10-15g)
Drinks	Drink plenty - aim for at least 6 - 8 cups/ mugs/glasses per day [2 litres].	○ 1 mug coffee/tea (200-250ml) ○ 'No added sugar' squash/fizzy drink ○ Water
Alcoholic Drinks	Up to 14 units a week for women Up to 21 units a week for men	1 unit of alcohol is: ○ ½ pint beer/lager/cider (4%) ○ 1 very small glass (80ml) of wine ○ 1 single pub measure of spirits
Salt	Try not to add salt to food. Keep processed/convenience food to a minimum	

Please note: 1 tsp = 1 teaspoon, 1tbsp = 1 tablespoon

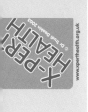

Dietary Action Plan - My Plan for Change

	Range of daily portions	Your present diet	Your goals	Approximate calories (Kcal) per portion
Starchy Carbohydrates	5-14			80
Fruit & Vegetables	5 - 9			50
Protein Foods	2 - 3			150
Milk & Dairy Foods	2 - 3			100
Fatty & Sugary Foods	0 - 4			100**

Drinks	6 - 8+			
Alcoholic Drinks <14 units for women / week <21 units for men / week	<2 units for women / day <3 units for men / day			100
Salt Added to Food Processed food	Keep to a minimum			------

** EXCEPT sugar/jam/honey which are around 50Kcal per portion

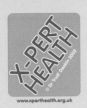

Setting A Goal:
Diet and Physical Activity

1. What is my biggest concern about my diet or physical activity levels?

_____

_____

2. Why am I concerned and what would the benefits be from addressing the concern?

_____

_____

3. What steps could I take to tackle the concern?

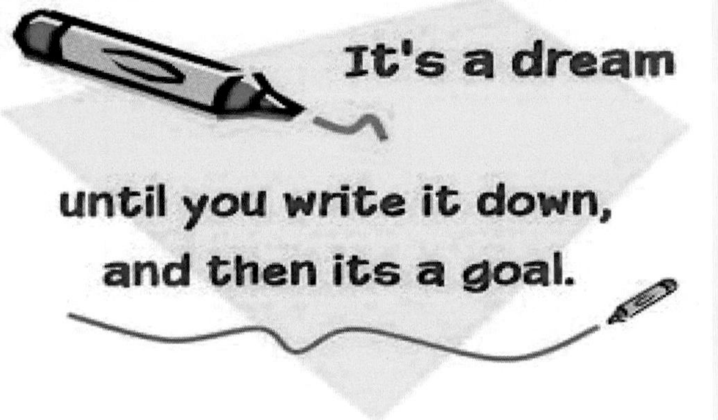

_____

_____

4. What is the first step I'm going to take?

What? _____

When? _____

Why? _____

It's a dream until you write it down, and then its a goal.

5. What happened? Did it work? How do I know?

_____

_____

How confident am I that I can make the first step? (circle)

0   1   2   3   4   5   6   7   8   9   10

not at all certain   totally certain

If you score below 7 - explore why ..... perhaps aim for a smaller goal!

Tick each day you achieve your goal and note comments

Monday _____

Tuesday _____

Wednesday _____

Thursday _____

Friday _____

Saturday _____

Sunday _____

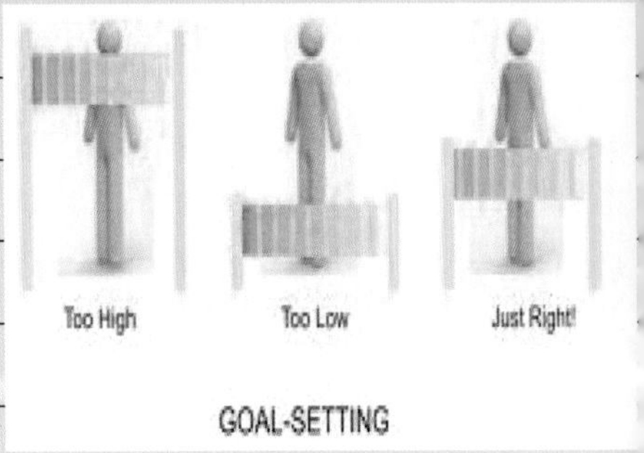

Too High   Too Low   Just Right!

GOAL-SETTING

Section 3: Carbohydrate ["Carb"] Awareness

Amount and Type of Carbohydrate

Increase your knowledge of "carbs" [starchy and sugary foods] and their effect on blood glucose levels. Become more skilful at estimating the amount of carbs you are eating.

Traditionally the 'sugar-free' diet was recommended for people with diabetes because it was assumed that sugary carbohydrates had a more rapid effect on blood glucose levels. Starchy carbohydrates such as bread, potatoes, rice and pasta were encouraged because it was assumed that they had a slow and long lasting effect on blood glucose levels. However, research has shown that it isn't quite as simple as this.

We now know that all starchy and sugary carbohydrate foods break down and release glucose into the blood at different rates and many starchy foods actually release glucose quicker than sugary foods. **The most important factor when considering blood glucose control is the AMOUNT of carbohydrate we eat.**

STARCH is made up from lots of units of glucose. Carbohydrate foods have different properties that allow them to digest and release glucose at different rates. Quick-releasing carbs are called high glycaemic index (GI) foods and slowly-releasing carbs, low GI foods. *How much carbohydrate you eat is the biggest factor that affects blood glucose but, once you know that you are eating the right amount of carbohydrate, swapping some quick releasing [high GI] carbs for slower releasing [low GI] carbs may also help to improve blood glucose levels.*

The guideline daily amount (GDA) for sugar is 90g [18 teaspoons] for women and 120g [24 teaspoons] for men. This may appear a lot but there are hidden sugars in many foods including natural-occurring foods such as fruit and milk and dairy food.

GLUCOSE is a simple unit, which is absorbed very quickly in the gut causing a rapid peak in blood glucose levels. SUCROSE, generally known as SUGAR is made from glucose and fructose. LACTOSE, is another type of sugar found in milk and milk products (MILK SUGAR). It is made up of glucose and galactose. Sucrose and lactose have less effect on blood glucose levels as they have to digest in the gut to release glucose. The released fructose and galactose is stored in the liver as a reserve energy source for between meals and during the night.

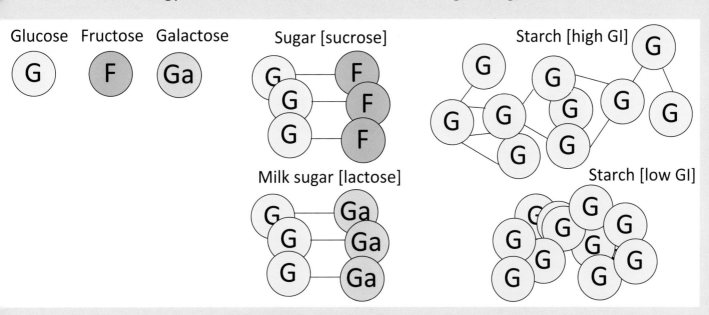

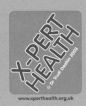
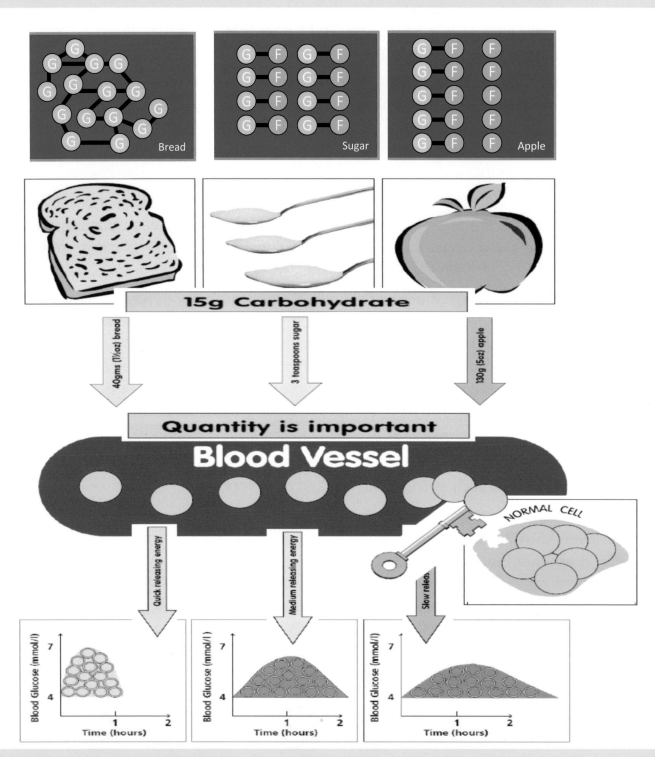

The guideline daily amount (GDA) for total carbohydrate is **230g for women and 300g for men.** This equates to 15 small slices of bread for women and 20 slices for men. However, this assumes that no other carbohydrates are eaten when in reality **all five food groups can contribute carbohydrate to the diet**.

Active people may require more than this and small or less active individuals, less. The brain requires 130g of glucose every day to function properly and therefore the **minimum amount has been set at 130g/day**. This also ensures that the diet doesn't become deficient in essential nutrients.

Carbohydrate Awareness

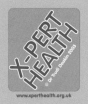

What is glucose? Carbohydrate foods (starchy and sugary) are building blocks of glucose. The food digests in the gut, breaking down and releasing glucose into the blood.

What is glucose used for in the body? Glucose is the preferred fuel for the body. The brain cannot function without a steady supply of glucose. It is therefore advisable that some carbohydrate food or drink is consumed on a regular basis.

Can I eat too many carbs? The amount of carbohydrate food and drink consumed is the most important factor in blood glucose control. Over-consuming carbohydrate food or drink will result in raised blood glucose levels. Becoming more carbohydrate aware can help you to control your diabetes. Portion sizes are important. A small inactive person is likely to require much less carbohydrate than a large active person.

Does it mean I can't eat sugar or desserts?

There is no special diet for people with diabetes. Sugar does not have a bigger impact on blood glucose levels than starch. Therefore, puddings, cake and chocolate can be eaten as part of a calorie controlled sensible eating plan:

- because the amount of carbs does affect blood glucose levels, you could *swap the carbohydrate* in the dessert for carbohydrate eaten elsewhere. For example, if you were having a pudding with the evening meal, you could reduce or cut out carbohydrate in the savoury course (potatoes/rice/pasta/bread) and just have the protein and vegetables/salad;

- if you inject insulin before each meal you could *learn how to adjust your insulin dose* according to the amount of carbohydrate eaten;

- you could eat the additional carbohydrate on a day when you are participating in more physical activity.

Refer to pages 43 to 46 to become more carbohydrate aware with 96 common foods. Remember that each small slice of bread contains 15g carbohydrate so consider each food in turn and question whether a portion of that food contains less carbohydrate than a slice of bread, the same quantity of carbohydrate or more carbohydrate. If it contains more carbohydrate, does it contain twice as much, three times as much or even more? This simple assessment will help you plan your diet and not eat too much carbohydrate.

> Just a word of caution: although we know that sweet carbohydrates do not affect blood glucose levels more than the same amount of savoury carbohydrates, it is not a good idea to swap them too often. Puddings, cakes and biscuits tend to contain more fat and calories and fewer vitamins and minerals than starchy carbohydrates such as bread, potato, rice and pasta. Therefore eating puddings, cakes and biscuits to excess could lead to weight gain and a deficiency in important nutrients such as vitamins and minerals.

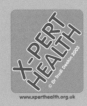

Glycaemic Index

Carbohydrate Food

HIGH GI
[quick-releasing]

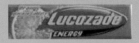

MEDIUM GI

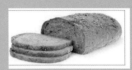

LOW GI
[slow-releasing]

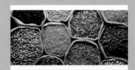

- Glucose / Lucozade
- Cornflakes / Rice Krispies
- Cheerios / Coco Pops
- Puffed Wheat / Rice cakes
- Bread (white/wholemeal)
- Rice (white & brown)
- Oatmeal biscuits / Scones
- Ryvita / Basmati rice
- Pitta breads / Chapatti
- New & Sweet potatoes
- Muesli / Porridge
- Sultana Bran / All-Bran
- Milk [semi-skimmed / soya]
- Fromage frais / Yoghurt
- Fruit / Vegetables
- Pulses [lentils / peas / beans]

- French bread / Crumpets
- Morning Coffee / Water biscuits
- Potatoes (baked/mashed/chips)
- Crispbread / Crackers
- Sugar / Jam / Fizzy drinks
- Shredded Wheat / Weetabix
- Rich Tea & Digestive biscuits
- Crisps / Popcorn / Muffins
- Breads (granary/wholegrain)
- Fruit & Fibre / Special K cereal
- Fruit loaf / Dried fruit
- Tinned fruit / Fruit juice
- Chocolate / Ice cream / Custard
- Pasta (fresh/dried)
- Rye/ Pumpernickel bread
- Baked beans / Dhal / Nuts

Carbohydrate foods and drinks that break down and release glucose more quickly are called HIGH GLYCAEMIC INDEX food and those which break down more slowly are called LOW GLYCAEMIC INDEX food.

Once you are happy that you are having the right amount of carbohydrate in the diet, changing the type of carbohydrate i.e. swapping some quick-releasing carbs for slower-releasing carbs, may have some extra benefits for helping to control blood glucose. For example, swapping a high GI cereal such as cornflakes for a low GI cereal such as porridge or replacing white/wholemeal bread for a multi-grain or multi-seed bread.

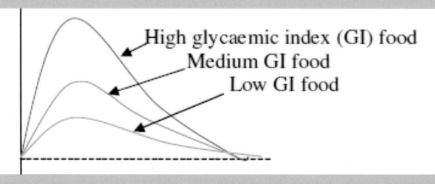

Please Note: Remember that although swapping high GI food for lower GI food will help to improve diabetes control, the key to achieving good blood glucose levels is in the AMOUNT of carbohydrates eaten.

Carbohydrate Awareness of Everyday Foods

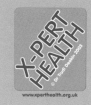

The darker the shading the higher the carbohydrate content, calories or glycaemic index [GI].

No carbohydrate (carbs) No glycaemic index (GI) Less than 10 calories	Low carbs (5g - 14g) Low GI Low Kcal (less than 100)	Moderate carbs (15g – 40g) Low to medium GI Moderate Kcal (100 - 300)
High carbs (41g - 60g) Medium to high GI High calories (301 - 500)	Very high carbs (> 60g) High GI Very high calories (> 500)	**Bread Equivalent** 0 - 4g = 0 slice 20g - 27g = 1 1/2 slices 5g-11g = 1/2 slice 28g - 35g = 2 slices 12g-19g = 1 slice > 36g = 2+ slices

Food and Serving	Bread Equivalent	Carb (g)	GI	Calories (Kcal)
All-Bran (50g) 7 tbsp – x 1 bowl	1 1/2	24	Low	139
Angel Delight 1/2 packet	1 1/2	20	Low / Medium	184
Apple Juice 200ml - x 1 small carton	1 1/2	20	Low	76
Apple x 1 medium (180g)	1 1/2	22	Low	90
Baked Beans - 210g (1/2 large tin)	1 1/2	26	Low	144
Banana – large 180g	3	42	Low / Medium	170
Basmati Rice (120g cooked)	2 1/2	38	Low / Medium	191
Carrot & Bean Soup - 1/2 tin (217g)	1	16	Low	84
Carrots (boiled) 2-3 tbsp (120g)	1/2	6	Low	29
Cauliflower - 2 tbsp (100g)	0	2	-	28
Chapatti x 2 110g	3	48	Low / Medium	258
Chick Peas (36g) - Cooked / 1 tablespoon	1/2	6	Low	43
Chips 180g (18 chips) (medium portion)	5	74	High	450
Chocolate Cake - 65g slice	2	35	Low	250
Chocolate-mini bar 21g	1	12	Low	109
- king size 100g	3 1/2	56	Low	520
Coca-Cola x 1 500ml bottle	3 1/2	54	Medium / High	215
Cornflakes (36g) 1 bowl (6 tbsp)	2	30	High	133
Crisps (30g) - x 1 packet	1	17	Low / Medium	181
Crumpet x 1	1 1/2	27	Medium / High	130

Carbohydrate Awareness of Everyday Foods

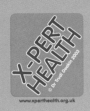

Food and Serving	Bread Equivalent	Carb (g)	GI	Calories (Kcal)
Custard - ½ tin (217g)	1 ½	23	Low	145
Date & Walnut Loaf - x 1 slice (50g)	1 ½	23	Low / Medium	127
Diet Coke (500ml bottle)	0	0	-	2
Digestive Biscuit x 2	1	18	Low / Medium	140
Dried Apricots x 6	1	14	Low	66
Fanta™ -x 1 bottle (500ml)	3 ½	52	Medium / High	215
Flavoured Milk - ½ bottle (250ml)	2	29	Low	175
French Bread 120g - 6" baguette	4 ½	66	High	324
Fruit Crumble & Custard	5	53	Medium	373
		23	Low	130
Total		Total = 76	Low / Medium	Total = 503
Granary Bread x 1 slice (45g)	1	19	Low / Medium	105
Grapefruit - ½ tin/200g (in natural juice)	1	15	Low	62
Grapefruit Juice x 1 glass (200ml)	1	18	Low	84
Grapes x 15 (100g)	1	12	Low	50
Hobnob (oat) biscuit x 2	1 ½	24	Low / Medium	190
Honey (20g) - 1 teaspoon	1	15	Low / Medium	58
Ice cream - x 1 scoop (50g)	1	12	Low / Medium	97
Jam – heaped teaspoon (15g)	½	10	Low / Medium	39
Jelly Babies x 5	1 ½	24	High	103
Lager x 1 can (500ml)	1	15	Medium / High	200
Lentil Soup - ½ tin (217g)	1	15	Low	81
Lentils - 2 tbsp (dry) (50g)	2	29	Low	159
Long Grain Rice ½ micro pk/120g cooked	2 ½	38	High	180
Lucozade - 1 x bottle (380ml)	4 ½		High	296
Malt Loaf (30g) - small slice	1	18	Low	86
Margarine 10g (2 teaspoons)	0	0	-	74
Mashed Potato- ½pk instant (250g cooked)	2	32	High	146

Carbohydrate Awareness of Everyday Foods

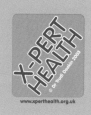

Food and Serving	Bread Equivalent	Carb (g)	GI	Calories (Kcal)
Melon - x 1 slice (200g)	½	8	Medium / High	38
Milk -1/3 pint (~200ml)	½	10	Low	98
Minced Beef 100g (cooked)	0	0	-	229
Muesli - medium bowl (70g = 5 x tablespoons)	3	42	Low / Medium	263
Muesli Bar Small	2	29	Low / Medium	212
Muller Light Yoghurt (1 pot)	1	17	Low	104
Mushy peas 2 tbsp (100g)	1 ½	20	Low	110
Naan bread - x 1 (130g)	4 ½	66	Medium / High	371
New Potatoes x 6 (200g boiled)	2	34	Medium / High	157
Oatcakes - x 2 (26g)	1	16	Low / Medium	115
Oatmeal (14g) x 1 tablespoon	½	9	Low / Medium	54
Old Potatoes (180g) - x 1 medium	3 ½	56	High	243
Orange (200g with skin) - x 1	1	13	Low	58
Orange Juice Sugar Free – bottle	0	3	Low / Medium	20
Orange Squash 50ml + 200ml water	1 ½	22	Medium / High	91
Peanuts - 100g packet	½	8	Low	622
Pears -1 small (100g)	1	14	Low	40
Peas (frozen) -2 tbsp	½	7	Low	52
Peas (tinned) - 2 tbsp (60g)	½	8	Low	48
Pitta Bread (60g) - x 1	2	32	Low / Medium	158
Pizza ½ 10"	5	70	Medium / High	600
Plums (86g) x 1 (small)	½	7	Low	31
Popcorn (plain) - x 1pk (100g)	3 ½	52	Medium	460
Pork Pie x 1 Individual 140g	2	35	Low / Medium	526
Porridge: 200ml milk + 3 tbsp oats (37g) Total	2 ½	10 27 Total = 37	Low	92 160 Total = 252
Red Kidney Beans - ½ small tin (60g)	½	10	Low	60

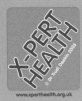

Carbohydrate Awareness
of Everyday Foods

Food and Serving	Bread Equivalent	Carb (g)	GI	Calories (Kcal)
Red wine 250ml- large glass	0	0.5	-	170
Rice Krispies x 7 tbsp (30g)	1 ½	26	High	114
Rice Pudding - ½ tin (217g)	2	30	Medium / High	162
Rich Tea Biscuits x 2	1	14	Low / Medium	88
Rye bread - 1 slice (96g)	1 ½	22	Low	105
Ryvita™ - x 2	1	12	Medium / High	50
Seeded bread - x 2 slices	2 ½	36	Low / Medium	264
Shortcake biscuits x 2	1	18	Medium / High	144
Shredded Wheat x 2	2	30	Medium / High	150
Spaghetti 125g uncooked weight+ tom sauce Total	5	64 / 10 / Total = 74	Low / Low / Total = Low	320 / 100 / Toatl = 420
Special K™ - x 1 bowl 36g (5tbsp)	1 ½	27	Low / Medium	133
Sugar - 2 tsp (10g)	½	10	Medium / High	40
Sultana Bran (50g) - 5 tbsp	1 ½	27	Low / Medium	130
Sultana Scone x 1	2	33	Medium / High	224
Sultanas – 40g heaped tablespoon	2	29	Low / Medium	122
Sweet Potato (140g cooked)	2 ½	39	Low / Medium	160
Sweetcorn (50g) - 2 tablespoons tinned	1	13	Low / Medium	62
Tinned Spaghetti - ½ tin (~200g)	1 ½	26	Low / Medium	122
Tomato ketchup - x 1 dollop (10g)	0	2.5	Medium / High	10
Tomatoes - x 2 (200g)	½	6	Low	33
Vegetable Oil (15g) - x 1 tbsp	0	0	-	135
Weetabix - x 2	1 ½	26	Medium / High	126
White sliced bread - 2 medium slices (80g)	2 ½	37	Medium / High	186
Wholemeal bread - 2 small slices (70g)	2	29	Medium / High	168
Yoghurt – SKI LF – x 1 pot (125g)	1 ½	20	Low	124

Carbohydrate Swap List

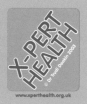

All food listed below has approximately 15g of carbohydrate in the portion sizes stated. Each one will release similar quantities of glucose into the blood as an average slice of bread.

Remember all carbohydrate food digests in our gut and is broken down into glucose. The glucose is then absorbed into the blood. We can measure our blood glucose. The normal range is between 4 – 7 mmol/l.

Carbohydrate Food	→	Digestion	→	Glucose	→	Blood glucose levels

FOOD	Weight of food	SWAP LIST Giving approx 15g of carbohydrate
Bread/toast	40g	1 medium slice
- Teacake - Bap - roll	40g	½ bap/roll
Cereal – Flakes (e.g. Cornflakes/Branflakes)	20g	2 - 3 tablespoons
- All Bran	40g	6 tablespoons
- Muesli	30g	2 tablespoons
- Weetabix/Shredded Wheat	20g	1 ½ biscuits
- Porridge oats	27g	2 tablespoons/1 sachet
Potato – baked (medium)	80g	1/3 small
- boiled	100g	2 egg-sized
- mashed	100g	1-2 level tablespoons
- chips	50g	4-6
Rice (cooked)	50g	1 heaped tablespoon
Pasta (cooked)	50g	2 tablespoons
Pulses – lentils, chick peas (cooked) baked beans	200g	2-3 tablespoons
Fruit - apple, orange, banana, pear, etc.	150g	1 small
- Grapefruit/mango	150g	½
- Grapes/cherries	80g	15
- Dried fruit	25g	1 tablespoon/small handful
- Fruit juice	150ml	small glass
Dairy Products – milk	300ml	½ pint
- Yoghurt (with artificial sweetener)	200g	1 medium pot
Sugar/jam/honey/syrup	15g	3 teaspoons sugar/1-2 teaspoons jam
Sweets – boiled/toffees	30g	2
- chocolate	30g	3-4 squares/1 fancy filled
Cake – plain/fruit loaf	30g	½ small slice
- bun/scone/mince pie	30g	½
Pudding – Christmas / chocolate brownie	30g	1 tablespoon/½ piece
- fruit crumble / trifle / tiramisu	50g	1 tablespoon
Biscuits – semi-sweet e.g. rich tea	20g	3
- digestive/oat	20g	1½
Crisps	30g	1 standard packet
Nuts	200g	1 medium packet

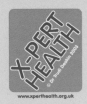

Setting a Goal:
How much carbohydrate am I eating?

Estimate how much carbohydrate you are eating on a daily basis.

Instructions:

1. Complete the carbohydrate awareness form on page 49 for a typical day estimating the carbohydrate consumed at each meal and snack. Refer to the 'Carbohydrate Awareness of Everyday Foods' tables and 'Carbohydrate Swap List' on pages 43 to 47.

2. Mark each carbohydrate with 'L' for low GI, 'M' for medium GI or 'H' for high GI.

3. Calculate the total number of carbohydrates consumed in the day.

Self-assessment: Are you happy with the amount and type of carbohydrate foods that you are having? What changes, if any would you like to make? For example: reducing the total daily intake of carbohydrate? Swapping high GI foods for low GI foods? Complete the goal setting form on page 50.

Daily Carbohydrate "Carbs" Intake – Sample	
Breakfast	Approx. Carbohydrate Content
- 4 tbsp muesli	40g (Low/Medium GI)
- 1 slice toast	15g (Medium/High GI)
- ½ teaspoon jam	5g (Medium GI)
- small glass fruit juice	15g (Low GI)
TOTAL	*75g*
Lunch	
- medium baked potato	65g (High GI)
- baked beans (small tin)	26g (Low GI)
- 1 pot yoghurt	17g (Low GI)
TOTAL	*108g*
Evening Meal	
3-4 tablespoons cooked spaghetti	40g (Low GI)
salad	-------
TOTAL	*40g*
Snacks: 1 fresh fruit	15g (Low GI)
20g chocolate bar	15g (Low GI)
milk in coffee/tea	10g (Low GI)
Supper: slice of fruit loaf	30g (Medium GI)
DAILY TOTAL	**293g**

← Average carbohydrate breakfast

← High carbohydrate lunch

← Low carbohydrate evening meal

A reminder about daily carbohydrate recommendations:
Minimum: 130g per day

Guideline Daily Amount (GDA): 230g (women) and 300g (man).

Please note:

Most people are consuming more carbohydrate than they think. Becoming more carbohydrate aware may help you control blood glucose levels and if desired, lose weight.

How much carbohydrate am I eating?

Breakfast	Carbohydrate content (g)
TOTAL	

Lunch	
TOTAL	

Evening Meal	
TOTAL	

Snacks: morning, afternoon & evening if consumed in addition to meals	

Supper:	

DAILY TOTAL	

Please note: you obtain carbohydrate from the following foods in addition to starchy and sugary foods: fruit; milk & yoghurt; pulses & nuts; fish and meat if breaded or battered.

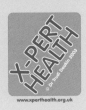

Setting A Goal: My Carb Intake

1. What is my biggest concern about my carbohydrate intake?

_____

_____

2. Why am I concerned and what would the benefits be from addressing the concern?

_____

_____

3. What steps could I take to tackle the concern?

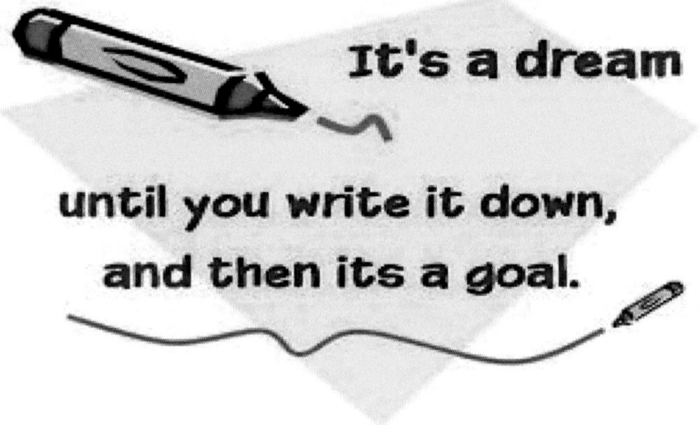

_____

_____

4. What is the first step I'm going to take?

What? _____

When? _____

Why? _____

It's a dream until you write it down, and then its a goal.

5. What happened? Did it work? How do I know?

_____

_____

How confident am I that I can make the first step? (circle)

0   1   2   3   4   5   6   7   8   9   10

not at all certain   totally certain

If you score below 7 - explore why ..... perhaps aim for a smaller goal!

Tick each day you achieve your goal and note comments

Monday   _____

Tuesday   _____

Wednesday _____

Thursday   _____

Friday   _____

Saturday   _____

Sunday   _____

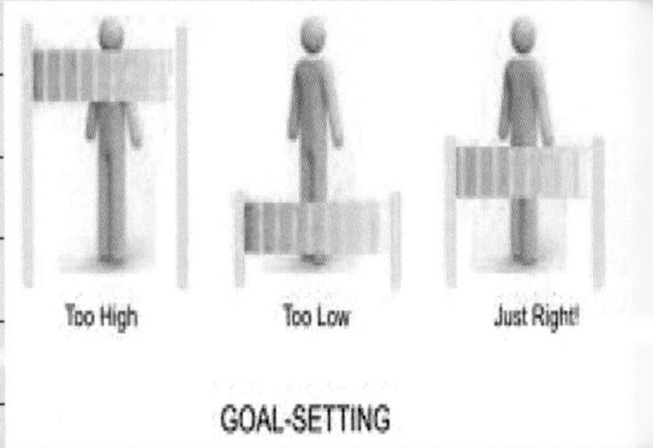

Too High   Too Low   Just Right!

GOAL-SETTING

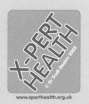

Section 4:
Reading and Understanding Food Labels

Read food labels by taking a closer look at food packaging.

1. The ingredients list

All ingredients in the product have to be listed in order of the greatest weight. Therefore, in the example shown [Tomato Soup], the ingredient with the highest content is 'Tomatoes' and lowest content 'Natural Flavouring".

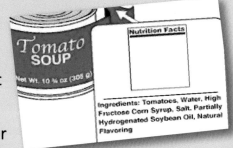

Individual ingredients can be listed under different names, for example, added sugars may be listed as sugar, sucrose, glucose, glucose syrup, invert syrup, maltose, fructose, lactose etc.

2. The nutritional information

A table will display the amount of each nutrient in that food. Some products will provide more

Nutrition	Per Slice 36g	Per 100g
Energy	89 kcal	248 kcal
Protein	3.7g	10.3g
Carbohydrate	16.7g	46.4g
of which sugars	1.2g	3.4g
Fat	0.9g	2.4g
of which saturates	0.3g	0.7g
Fibre	1.3g	3.7g
Sodium	0.15g	0.41g
Equivalent as salt	0.38g	1.05g

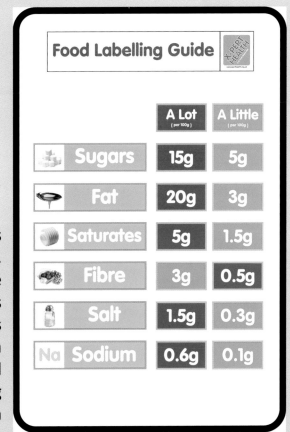

Above is a sample table for granary bread. Many products display nutritional information *per 100g* and *per serving*. The amount *per serving* is useful if you eat the recommended serving size. The *per 100g* allows comparison with different products/brands. It also helps you identify whether a food or drink contains 'a lot' or 'a little' sugar, fat, saturates, fibre and salt by referring to food labelling guides. A Food Labelling Guide with a magnifying glass (so you can read the label!) may be purchased from the X-PERT online shop at www.xperthealth.org.uk.

Each serving contains

Calories	Fat	Saturates	Sugars	Salt
300	7.7g	2.0g	42.2g	2.0g
15%	11%	10%	47%	33%

of your guideline daily amount

3. Guideline Daily Amount (GDA) Labelling

This labelling system can be found on some food packaging. It states the amount of calories, sugar, total fat, saturated fat and salt that can be found in a serving. It also presents what proportion (%) of your guideline daily amount (GDA) there is in a serving.

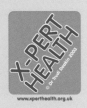

Reading and Understanding Food Labels

The GDAs for calories, sugars, fat, saturates and salt are based on daily recommendations for an average adult or child of healthy weight and average activity levels. To keep things simple, the labelling system on food packaging is based on the GDAs for women.

	Calories	Carbohydrate	Sugars	Fat	Saturates	Fibre	Salt
							Less than
Men	2500	300g	120g	95g	30g	24g	6g
Women	2000	230g	90g	70g	20g	24g	6g
Children (aged 5 -10)	1800	220g	85g	70g	20g	15g	4g

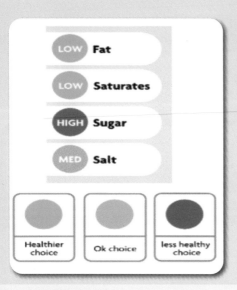

4. Traffic light labelling

Many foods have traffic light labelling to help you to see how healthy or unhealthy a food may be and making the comparison between different products or brands much easier.

The traffic light colours are used for amounts of fat, saturated fat, sugar and salt per serving.

Most foods will be labelled with a mixture of the 3 colours, so when comparing similar foods try to choose those with more green and amber lights and fewer red lights.

5. Confusing?

One downfall is that the GDA and Traffic Light labelling systems on the *front of package* does not include total carbohydrates and therefore is not as helpful to people with diabetes who wish to count carbohydrate. To obtain that information the consumer will have to read the nutritional table which is normally found on the *back of package*. The sample table for pizza informs the consumer that there are 44g carbs per 1/2 pizza.

NUTRITION			GDA	
Typical values	per 100g	per ½ pizza	adult	per ½ pizza
Energy kJ	815	1475		
Energy kcal	195	355	2000	18%
Protein	9.2g	16.7g	45g	37%
Carbohydrate	24.2g	43.8g	230g	19%
of which sugars	4.6g	8.3g	90g	9%
Fat	6.7g	12.1g	70g	17%
of which saturates	2.8g	5.1g	20g	26%
Fibre	2.4g	4.3g	24g	18%
Sodium	0.54g	0.98g	2.4g	41%
Equivalent as salt	1.35g	2.45g	6g	41%
GDA = Guideline daily amount				

Remember there are no good and bad foods.
Foods that are high in fat, sugar or salt can be eaten in small amounts as part of a healthy balanced diet.

Some foods have a red traffic light but may be beneficial for health
For example, oily fish has a red light for fat but it is a good source of omega-3 fats that are good for heart health. Fruit and milk products are health promoting and their consumption is important to ensure adequate intake of vitamins, minerals, fibre and calcium. However, they are naturally high in sugars such as sucrose, fructose and lactose and will display an amber or red light for sugar. Therefore, do not omit these foods and instead check the nutritional table on the back of package to assess the total carbohydrate content per serving.

Nutritional Claims / Food Tips

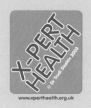

NUTRITIONAL CLAIMS	WHAT DO THEY MEAN?
Fat free/sugar free	Contains very small amounts of fat or sugar [less than 0.5g per 100g]. Be careful: they may have additional calories from other sources!
Low fat Less than 5% fat	Contains *less than 3g fat per 100g* of product [less than 3%] The food contains less than 5g fat per 100g. Be careful: it may still be high fat if eaten in excessive amounts.
Reduced fat/sugar	Contains *at least 30% less fat/sugar* than its regular comparable product. Be careful: it does not necessarily mean the product is low fat/sugar. For example reduced fat crisps still have 23g fat per 100g.
No added sugar	*No sugar has been added to the product.* When looking at a label it may still show the sugar content to be high but this will be natural sugars for example, in fruit juice and yoghurt. Be careful: all sugars [natural or added] release glucose into the blood.
80 to 97% fat free	Be careful: It can be misleading suggesting that the product is healthier than it is! If a product is 80% fat free, *it still contains 20% fat*.
Diabetic Foods	Diabetes UK has advised that labelling foods as "Diabetic" or "Suitable for diabetics" should be stopped. such foods are often more expensive and may lead some people to believe they may have a stamp of approval and are beneficial or even essential for people with diabetes. There is no need to purchase diabetic foods.

Food Group	Portion Size	Why it is good to eat	Recommendations
STARCHY CARBOHYDRATES	The amount of carbs you eat is a key factor in blood glucose control	Carbohydrate is our preferred energy source but remember it all breaks down into glucose. *Over-consuming starchy foods will result in high blood glucose levels.*	Have a daily intake of wholegrains.
BREAD wholegrain multigrain multi-seed raisin bread pitta bread fruit teacakes	1 slice bread 1/2 pitta 1/2 teacake	Low in fat. Try varieties with added fibre such as wholegrain, granary, oats and seeds. These varieties help to prevent and treat constipation. *Wholegrains help heart health, blood glucose control and weight management.*	
POTATOES new old mashed	100g potato 2 to 3 new 1/2 old 1 to 2 level tablespoons	A good source of vitamin C. New and sweet potatoes release glucose more slowly than old potatoes. *Overconsumption of potato and chips results in high blood glucose.*	
CEREALS any containing oats, nuts or fruit e.g. porridge/ muesli/All Bran Sultana Bran	1 bowl (2 to 4 tablespoons)	Try varieties with added fibre such as wholegrain, oats, nuts and seeds. These varieties have a lower glycaemic index. *These help to prevent constipation and make you feel fuller for longer.*	
pasta basmati rice	1 to 2 tablespoons	Pasta releases glucose into the blood at a slower rate than bread or potatoes. Basmati rice is slower releasing than other types of rice. *Over consumption leads to high blood glucose levels.*	

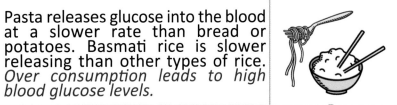

Food Tips

Food Group	Portion Size	Why it is good to eat	Recommendations
FRUIT & VEG • apple/orange • mango/melon • banana • grapes • dried fruit • figs/apricots • dates • tinned fruit • fruit juice • vegetables • salad	1 small 1/2 mango/slice 1 small handful (15) handful (25g) 3 to 4 3 to 4 1/2 tin 1 glass (150ml) 2 to 3 tbs 1 bowl	Fat free. Excellent source of anti-oxidants, vitamins and minerals. Slow-release energy. Ensure variety by choosing a range of colours. Reduce carbohydrate load by choosing tinned fruit in natural juice. Only 1 glass of fruit juice can be counted as 1 portion as it lacks fibre and is concentrated in carbohydrate. *Protection against heart disease and cancer.*	5 to 9 portions per day 1 portion = 80g
PROTEIN FOODS <u>Oily Fish</u> salmon/mackerel pilchards/sardines herring/fresh tuna kippers/trout <u>Seafood</u> prawns mussels <u>White Fish</u> cod/haddock plaice/whiting <u>Meat</u> lean meat and poultry <u>Pulses</u> lentils, peas & beans <u>Eggs</u> <u>Nuts & Seeds</u>	Oily fish: 100g White fish and seafood 120-140g Meat: 85g Poultry: 100g 2 to 4 tablespoons 2 eggs (100g) 2 tablespoons	*Omega-3 fatty acids help to reduce heart disease and decrease pain and morning stiffness with arthritis.* Choose fresh / smoked / tinned [in tomato sauce, brine or water as oil adds unnecessary fat and calories]. Seafood is low in fat and an excellent source of the antioxidant, selenium. White fish is a good source of protein and is low in fat. Watch out for hidden fat when breaded, battered or served with cream or cheese sauces. Red meat is a good source of iron. Many lean meats are less than 5% fat. *If eaten to excess may reduce glucose tolerance.* Pulses are an excellent source of soluble fibre. Be aware of added fat in dhal. *Good source of protein.* High in fibre and a good source of monounsaturated fat.	Protein: 2 to 3 portions per day Oily fish: maximum of 4 portions per week for boys, men and post-menopausal women. Maximum of 2 portions a week for girls, pregnant or breast-feeding women. Red meat: less than 500g per week. Up to 7/week.
MILK & DAIRY FOODS skimmed/semi-skimmed milk cottage/half-fat cheese low fat/virtually fat free yoghurt	1/3 pint milk 1 small carton/ 30g chunk 150/200g carton	Slow release energy. All products listed are reduced in animal fat [saturates] and calories. Some low fat cheeses are also low in saturates and high in monounsaturated fat (Super Light). Yoghurt can be a healthy snack or dessert. *Good source of calcium for healthy teeth and bones.*	2 or 3 portions per day.
SUGARY FOODS sugar jam / honey half-spoon sugar artificial sweetener	2 teaspoons	Sugar provides carbs and calories but no other nutrients. 1 teaspoon = 5g carbs & 20 calories. 1 teaspoon = 10g carbs & 40 calories. 1 teaspoon = 2.5g carbs & 10 calories. 1 teaspoon = 0 carbs & 0 calories.	Use sparingly. fatty & sugary foods 0 to 4 portions per day.

Food Tips

Food Group	Portion Size	Why it is good to eat	Recommendations
FATS & OILS olive oil rapeseed oil vegetable oil Utterly Butterly Bertolli	10 ml oil [Be careful – all fats contain the same amount of calories]. 2 teaspoons spread (14g) [Choose low fat spreads to reduce calories].	*Monounsaturated fat is the preferred fat for heart health* It reduces the bad (LDL) cholesterol and is less prone to oxidation. Good sources include olive and rapeseed vegetable oils & spreads; and nuts. Polyunsaturated fat [e.g. sunflower, safflower, sesame, soya, corn, linseed and grapeseed oils] also reduce LDL cholesterol but are more prone to oxidation leading to cell damage.	Use sparingly: 0 to 4 portions per day.
HEALTHIER SNACKS or DESSERTS popcorn malt loaf dried fruits natural nuts Angel Delight milk puddings fruit crumble ice cream frozen yoghurt	 Small bowl (25g) 1 slice (25g) handful (25g) handful (25g) 1/4 sachet made-up (75ml) small bowl (50g) 1 scoop (40g)	*These release glucose more slowly than bread but watch portion sizes and consider substituting for other carbs.* Can add less salt if made at home. High fibre, low fat. Good source of iron. High fibre, high in monounsaturates. Use the 'no added sugar' version and make-up with skimmed milk. Save carbs & cals: use skimmed milk and artificial sweetener. Make crumble with monounsaturated spread and add oats. Read nutritional information label to choose varieties that have fewer calories, fat and carbs.	
DRINKS fruit juices and no added sugar squash/cordial	1 small glass (150ml)	Fruit juices are a concentrated form of carbohydrate and not as nutritious as fruit. 'No added sugar' squashes contain virtually no carbohydrate or calories.	Juice: up to x1 glass per day Fluid: at least 6-8 glasses/day
ALCOHOL	1 unit: = 1/2 pint beer or lager. = 25ml measure of spirits. = 1 small (80ml) glass of wine. .... 1 large (250ml) glass of wine is 3 units. A standard 12% bottle of wine (750ml) contains 9 units.	Try not to drink on an empty stomach. Keep within healthy limits of alcohol. Spread alcohol intake over the week. Have alcohol free days. Mixers – use sugar-free soft drinks to reduce carbohydrate load. Be aware: low carbohydrate beers are high in alcohol. Be aware: sweet sherry, liqueurs, sweet ciders & alcopops can be high in carbs. Be aware: low alcohol beers can be high in carbs. All types of alcoholic drinks are high in calories. *Consuming a small amount of alcohol can be beneficial to health.*	Men = up to 21 units/week Women = up to 14 units/week

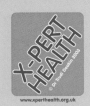

Reading Nutritional Labels

Information that can be obtained from reading the nutritional label on food packaging

Fruit & Vegetables	
1. A high fibre vegetable	Garden peas [5g fibre per 100g]
2. The number of grapes providing 15g carbohydrate	~ 15 [1 grape is approx. 1g carb]
3. A fruit that contains less than 10g carbs per 100g	Strawberries [6g carbs per 100g]
4. A fruit that contains more than 50g carbs per 100g	Sultanas [69g carbs per 100g]
Starchy Carbohydrates	
5. A bread that contains 15-20g carbs per slice	Hovis Seed Sensations™[18.5g/slice]
6. A cereal that is high in soluble fibre	Porridge oats[1.8g per 45g]
7. A cereal that contains more than 10g fibre per portion	All Bran™ [11g per 40g]
8. A cereal that contains less than 1g fibre per portion	Cornflakes™ [0.9g per 30g]
9. A food that contains more than 40g carbs per portion	Pasta [50g per 75g uncooked]
Protein Foods	
10. A protein food that contains carbohydrate	Chicken Kievs [17g per 150g]
11. A protein food that is low in saturated fat	Pork Lion Fillets [1.1g per 120g]
12. A protein food that is low fat	Prawns [0.3g per 100g]
13. A protein food that contains monounsaturated fat	Beef steak [3.8g per 100g]
14. An oily fish containing omega-3 fats	Salmon Fillets [4.4g per 190g]
15. A protein food that is high in soluble fibre	Baked Beans [7.9g per 200g]
Milk & Dairy Foods	
16. A high fat dairy food	Cheddar cheese [10.3g per 30g]
17. A low fat milk & dairy food	Muller Light yoghurt™ [0.2g/200ml]
18. A low saturated fat cheese	Cottage cheese [0.7g per 76g]
19. A high monounsaturated fat cheese	SuperLite™ [3.3g per 30g]
20. A dairy food that may reduce LDL [bad] cholesterol	Benecol Light™ [2g stanol/67.5g]
Fatty & Sugary Foods	
21. A spread high in monounsaturated fat	Utterly Butterly™ [28.8g per 100g]
22. A spread high in saturated fat	Butter [54g per 100g]
23. An oil that is high in monounsaturated fat	Olive oil [73g per 100g]
24. An oil that is high in polyunsaturated fat	Flora™ [58g per 100g]
25. A chocolate bar that contains 25g carbs	45g Cadbury Dairy Milk™ bar
26. A bag of crisps that contains 180 calories	34.5g Walkers™ crisps
Drinks	
27. A low fat hot chocolate drink	Highlights™ [1.4g fat per portion]
28. A recommended drink to treat hypoglycaemia	Lucozade™ [Glucose 86g/500ml]
Alcoholic Drinks	
29. A can of lager that contains 2 units of alcohol	500ml can [4% alcohol]
Salt	
30. A food that is high in salt	Salami [1g per 31.3g portion]

Fat Awareness

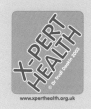

Fat is the greatest source of calories in the diet. Butter, spreads and oils are visible fats. However, most foods contain *hidden fats* because we can't see them. There are five types of dietary fat.

Saturated fat: Found in: fatty cuts of meat; butter, cheese & cream; chocolate, biscuits, cakes & pastries. It is used to make bad [LDL] cholesterol and if we eat too much of it, the excess LDL cholesterol causes insulin resistance and also forms fatty plaques and clogs up blood vessels, increasing the risk of heart disease. The average man should eat no more than 30g a day and a woman, no more than 20g a day. The less the better!

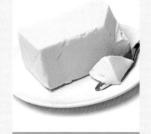

Butter

Trans fat: This is harmful because it acts in the body as saturated fat and raises LDL cholesterol, increases insulin resistance, waist circumference and the risk of heart disease. High-fat baked goods (especially doughnuts, cookies, cakes, chips and crackers) and deep-fried foods are more likely to contain hydrogenated fat that gives rise to trans fats. Those most at risk from trans fats are people eating deep-fried takeaway food regularly and/or purchasing cheaper or foreign brands of processed food.

Cakes, Burgers and Chips

Dietary cholesterol: Found in animal products such as eggs, liver, kidneys and shellfish. We now know that diets high in saturated fat have a far greater impact on LDL cholesterol levels and associated health risks than the intake of dietary cholesterol. *What are the recommendations for the number of eggs permitted each week?* Two eggs = 1 portion of protein. Eggs also contain saturated fat and therefore 7 or more eggs a week may increase risk of heart disease.

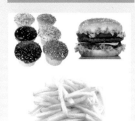

Eggs

Polyunsaturated fat: Found in oils like sunflower, safflower, sesame, corn & soya; oily fish such as salmon, mackerel and sardines; nuts and seeds such as walnuts, brazil nuts; sunflower & sesame seeds. It is essential for health because it cannot be made by the human body. Omega-3 fats are recognised for their protective effect on heart health. However, these fats are less stable when heated and can lead to cell damage. Therefore it is not advisable to eat more that 10% of calories i.e. 20g/day for women and 30g/day for men and it is better to have sources of omega-3 polyunsaturates.

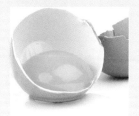

Sunflower Oil

Monounsaturated fat: Good sources include olive and rapeseed oil [many vegetable oils are pure rapeseed oil), Bertolli™, Utterly Butterly™. It is also found in peanut or groundnut oil; and in nuts such as peanuts, almonds, cashews, brazil nuts. Monounsaturated fat reduces the lethal LDL cholesterol levels and is more stable, protecting the body cells from damage. It is the best option for people with diabetes.

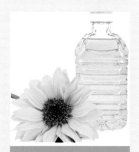

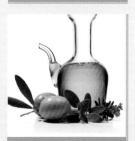

Olive Oil

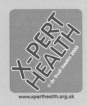

Comparing Foods

Meat: not all red meat is high in saturated fat. Some cuts contain less than 5% fat and half of this fat is monounsaturated fat, a better fat for the heart because it doesn't increase the LDL [bad] cholesterol.

However, fatty and processed red meat increase insulin resistance and risk of heart disease.

Type of red meat	Total fat/100g	Saturated fat/100g
Pork loin fillet [lean]	2.9	1.1
Roasted lean topside beef	3.2	1.5
Beef steak	8.2	3.3
Lean beef steak mince	11.5	5.1
Dry cured back bacon	17.7	6.9
Pork sausages	18.3	6.5
Beef mince	28.0	12.7
Salami	51.3	21.0

Cheese: if you are a cheese lover you can now purchase a low fat variety with a much lower saturated fat content. It tastes good too!

Nutrient per 100g	Super Light™	Cheddar
Calories	280 kcal	410 kcal
Protein	30g	25g
Fat	17g	**34g**
Saturates	1g	**22g**
Mono fat	11g	11g
Poly fat	5g	1g
Omega-3	2g	0g
Carbs	3g	0g
Calcium	909mg	721mg

Omega-3: eating 1 or 2 portions of oil-rich fish per week is advisable as it will provide around 2-4g of omega-3 fatty acids. Current average intake in the UK falls short of the recommendation. If you don't like oily fish, the table below provides alternative sources.

Omega 3 special products	Serving	Omega-3
Probiotic drink	100 ml	0.8g
Eggs	1 egg	1.25g
Fish fingers	3	1.5g
Spread	10g/2tsp	0.28g
Seven Seas™ (Extra high strength)	1 capsule	11g
	10ml oil	2.3g

Spreads: Butter contains the greatest amount of saturated fat. People with diabetes and/or heart disease are advised to have spreads that contain more monounsaturates. Trans fats have been removed from spreads in the UK.

Fat	Butter	Flora™	Bertolli™	Utterly Buterly™	Olive Light
Total	82%	59%	59%	49%	38%
Saturates	56g	12g	14g	13g	9g
Polyunsaturates	3g	30g	15g	10g	6g
Monounsaturates	20g	17g	30g	24g	21g

Focus on Alcohol

Recommendations: Men should drink no more than 21 units of alcohol per week [and no more than four units in any one day]. Women should drink no more than 14 units of alcohol per week [and no more than three units in any one day].

Drinking 1 to 2 units per day may be beneficial for health by helping to protect from heart disease. However, the more you drink above the safe limits, the more harmful alcohol is likely to be and it can lead to liver disease, pancreatitis, erectile dysfunction, high blood pressure, depression, damage to nerve tissue, cancer, obesity and addiction.

Beer and Lager per pint (568ml)	Alcohol units	Calories (kcal)	Carbs (g)
Ale, brown	2.7	227	17
Ale, strong	2.8	244	35
Guinness (draught)	2.3	210	18
Beer, Bitter	2	182	13
Foster's lager (4%)	2.3	170	18
Carling lager (draught 5%)	2.8	244	8
Alcohol free Becks (0.05%)	0.3	114	28
Light Corona (4.5%)	2.6	182	0
Wine per glass (250ml)	Alcohol units		Carbs (g)
Wine, red (12%)	3	170	1
Wine, rose (12%)	3	178	6
Wine, white, dry (12%)	3	185	2
Wine, white, med (12%)	3	185	9
Wine, white, sweet (12%)	3	229	15
Spirits per pub measure (25ml)	Alcohol units		Carbs (g)
Whisky	1	56	0
Gin	1	56	0
Alcopops per bottle (275ml)	Alcohol units		Carbs (g)
Smirnoff Ice	1.1	157	33

The table above provides alcohol units, calorie and carbohydrate guidance for a range of drinks. If you would like to calculate your weekly average, you may find it useful to visit the following website that provides an automated alcohol unit and calorie calculator: http://www.drinkaware.co.uk/tips-and-tools/drink-diary/

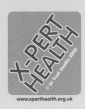

Setting A Goal: The Foods I Buy

1. What is my biggest concern about the foods I buy?

_____

_____

2. Why am I concerned and what would the benefits be from addressing the concern?

_____

_____

3. What steps could I take to tackle the concern?

_____

_____

4. What is the first step I'm going to take?

What? _____

When? _____

Why? _____

It's a dream until you write it down, and then its a goal.

5. What happened? Did it work? How do I know?

_____

_____

How confident am I that I can make the first step? (circle)

0   1   2   3   4   5   6   7   8   9   10

not at all certain   totally certain

If you score below 7 - explore why ..... perhaps aim for a smaller goal!

Tick each day you achieve your goal and note comments

Monday _____

Tuesday _____

Wednesday _____

Thursday _____

Friday _____

Saturday _____

Sunday _____

Too High   Too Low   Just Right!

GOAL-SETTING

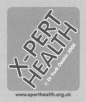

Hyperglycaemia

What does it mean?

Blood Vessel

Hyperglycaemia is raised blood glucose levels:
- above 7 mmol/l before meals
- above 8.5 mmol/l two hours after meals

Possible symptoms of hyperglycaemia:
- tiredness and lethargy
- warm, sweaty
- dry mouth, thirsty
- frequent urination (especially at night)
- urinary infections
- impaired healing
- blurred vision

Treatment: lifestyle review & medication

Prevention
- Watch those carbohydrate portions
- Be as active as you can
- Lose weight if required
- Don't forget to take your medication
- Take insulin/diabetes tablets as prescribed
- If you are ill continue with medication

Hypoglycaemia

What does it mean?

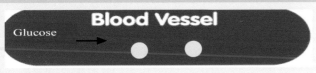

Glucose **Blood Vessel**

Hypos occur when the blood glucose level drops too low, below 4 mmol/l.

Possible symptoms of hypoglycaemia:
- shaking, sweating
- confusion, tingling
- headache, slurred speech
- mood changes, irritability
- blurred vision, unsteadiness
- hunger, drowsiness
- unsteadiness, drowsiness

Prevention
- Eat regular meals
- Eat some carbohydrate at each meal
- Eat more carbohydrate if more active
- Take your diabetes tablets/insulin correctly
- Don't drink alcohol on an empty stomach
- Adjust insulin in hot weather
- Have a diabetes and medication review

Treatment

ACTION	WHAT	DETAIL
STEP 1	Take 15-20g rapid acting carbohydrate	A glass (100ml) of Lucozade™ (17g glucose) OR 4 x Glucotab™ glucose tablets (16g glucose) OR 6 x Dextro Energy™ dextrose tablets (18g glucose)
STEP 2	Have meal or snack containing 2-3 portions of carbohydrate	1 portion is: 1 slice of bread 2 egg-sized potatoes 2 digestive biscuits 1 piece of fruit/15 grapes
STEP 3	Monitor blood glucose	Ensure blood glucose is above 4 mmol/l and do not drive or operate machinery for 45 minutes after the blood glucose levels return to normal.

6

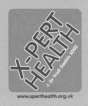

Possible Complications

Possible Longer-Term Complications		What does it mean?
Stroke section of the brain becomes starved of blood and oxygen	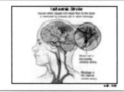	Raised blood pressure, blood glucose and blood cholesterol can damage and narrow the blood vessels. Part of the brain then becomes starved of blood and oxygen.
Retinopathy damage to the eyes	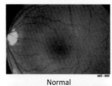 Normal / Retinopathy	Damage to the tiny blood vessels at the back of the eye is caused as a result of raised blood glucose & blood pressure levels. Good control is the key to prevention. It is vital to have an annual eye check where a digital camera is used to take a picture. If damage is found, laser treatment can be very effective at sealing the leaky blood vessels and preventing the damage from getting worse.
Gingivitis and periodontitis gum disease	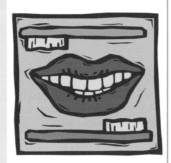	Although anyone can get gum disease, it is estimated that people with diabetes can be up to three times more likely to develop it. Gum disease can range from gingivitis, which causes red, swollen, painful gums which bleed easily, to periodontitis where there is damage to the tissue surrounding the teeth and bone loss which can lead to tooth loss. A dentist or hygienist will be able to advise on the best brushing methods to keep any gum problems under control.
Hypertension raised blood pressure	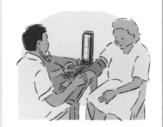	Blood pressure guidelines are stricter for people with diabetes because the combination of raised blood glucose and blood pressure can lead to the damage of blood vessels. Target blood pressure is a reading below 140/80 although if there is any damage to the eyes or kidneys, a stricter reading below 130/80 is recommended. 24-hour monitoring is often required to confirm the diagnosis.
Coronary Heart Disease [CHD] heart muscle starved of blood & oxygen	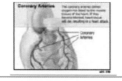	Raised blood pressure, blood glucose and blood cholesterol can damage the blood vessels in the heart. Heart muscle becomes starved of blood and oxygen.
Cardiovascular Disease [CVD] collection of heart & blood vessel problems	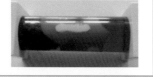	CVD is not a single condition but a general term used to describe conditions affecting the heart and blood vessels such as unhealthy cholesterol levels [dyslipidaemia].
Atherosclerosis hardening of the arteries [blood vessels]	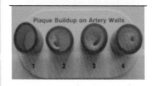	Risk factors include: fat deposits of LDL [bad] cholesterol that build up on the walls of the arteries; smoking; high blood pressure; raised blood glucose levels; being overweight and inactivity.

Possible Complications

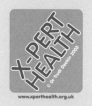

Possible Longer-Term Complications		Definitions
Angina chest pain		Angina is an uncomfortable feeling or pain in the chest. It is caused by damaged blood vessels not being able to deliver enough oxygen to heart muscle.
Nephropathy kidney damage		Kidney damage occurs when raised blood pressure and blood glucose levels damage the tiny blood vessels that supply the kidneys. Damage to the filtering system results in protein leaking into the urine.
Autonomic Neuropathy damage to the nerves that perform automatic functions		Damage to the nerves in the gut and sex organs can result in nausea, bloating, diarrhoea, constipation, erectile dysfunction, vaginal dryness and reduced ability to orgasm.
Peripheral Vascular Disease damage to blood vessels in the arms and legs		Fatty deposits build up in the arteries (blood vessels) in the arms or legs. This results in blood flow being restricted to the arm and leg muscles.
Sensory Neuropathy damage to the nerves that allow us to feel with our hands and feet		Diabetes can cause nerve damage to legs /feet (sometimes arms/hands) resulting in reduced sensation (numbness), tingling and/or pain. Daily foot care is important (page 64) and feet should be checked regularly for signs of injury or wounds.
Foot Ulcers damage to the feet due to poor circulation and reduced sensation		Raised blood glucose and poor circulation prevent enough oxygen and nutrients healing a wound and ulceration of the foot may result. Preventable with good daily foot care.

Prevention

○ Obtain target blood glucose levels as often as possible.
○ Achieve blood pressure control.
○ Monitor blood cholesterol levels.
○ Lose weight if necessary.
○ Watch your alcohol intake.
○ Stop or reduce smoking.
○ Use monounsaturates oils and spread.
○ Reduce saturated (animal) fat.
○ Increase physical activity levels, aiming for 30-60 minutes each day.
○ Eat more fruit and vegetables, aiming for at least five portions each day.
○ Eat more wholegrains, soluble fibre and less processed food.
○ Take medication as prescribed.

> **IMPORTANT:** Complications of diabetes are largely PREVENTABLE. Understanding what they are and how they may be prevented is important. The information isn't meant to frighten you but to help you look after your long-term health and quality of life.

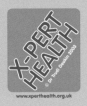

Taking Care of Feet with Diabetes

Foot problems can affect anyone who has diabetes becuase they are more likely to have poor circulation and reduced feeling in the feet. It is important to understand how they develop and how they can be prevented or detected early so that they can be treated successfully.

How do foot problems develop?

Diabetes, particularly if poorly controlled, can damage nerves in your feet and legs. This is called neuropathy. *Sensory neuropathy* affects the nerves that tell us how we feel temperature and pain. You could injure your feet without realising it and if not treated properly, they injury could become infected or develop into an ulcer. *Motor neuropathy* affects the nerves responsible for movements, such as walking and could cause your feet to alter shape. Your toes may become clawed (curled) and occasionally a serious condition known as a Charcot Foot can develop, a condition where the foot becomes hot, swollen and inflamed. *Autonomic neuropathy* affects the nerves which work the sweat glands resulting in dry and cracked feet.

Diabetes, high blood pressure, a high saturated fat diet and smoking may also affect the circulation by clogging up the arteries that supply blood, oxygen and nutrients to the feet.

How can they be prevented?

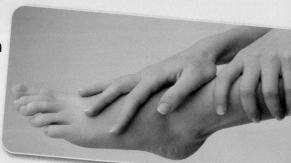

- Wash your feet daily, testing the temperatures with your elbow to avoid scalding accidents.
- Never soak your feet as this can lead to dry and cracked skin.
- Dry your feet particularly between your toes to reduce the risk of fungal infections.
- Cut toe nails according to the shape of your toe.
- Avoid cutting down the side of the nail as you could develop in-growing toe nails. It's easier to cut toe nails after bathing or washing.
- Never use sharp instruments on your feet and check the insides of shoes for ridges.
- Apply moisturiser to keep your skin supple and prevent cracking.
- Avoid walking in bare feet as you may stand on something sharp and not notice.
- Check your feet daily for injuries. If you cannot reach your feet then use a mirror or get someone else to look.
- Buy shoes that are: broad fitting with deep and rounded toe area; flat or low heeled; fastened by a lace/buckle; soft leather with as few seams as possible. Have feet measured.
- Do not treat corns or callouses yourself or use corn plasters as they contain acid. Seek advice from your practice nurse, GP or podiatrist.
- Make sure feet are not exposed to extremes of temperature. On holiday take comfortable well-fitting shoes that are not new. On long journeys do foot exercises to improve circulation. Avoid walking barefoot on beaches and pavements as this can cause burns.
- Achieve good control of blood glucose, blood pressure and blood cholesterol levels.
- Reduce saturated (animal) fat, take regular physical activity and stop smoking.
- Change socks and stockings daily and choose natural fibres such as cotton rather than nylon. Ladies should avoid wearing tight hosiery which restrict blood flow to feet.

How can they be detected early?

Make sure you get your annual foot check by a trained healthcare professional who will check the pulses in the feet and lower leg to assess blood flow and also use instruments to check the sensations in the feet.

Looking After My Diabetes: Annual Review

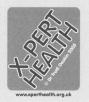

It is important to remember that your diabetes annual review is to enable you to lead a normal and healthy life. The following should be checked at least once a year:

- Blood glucose control [HbA1c]
- Kidney function: [ACR or eGFR]
- Blood fats [Total cholesterol, LDL, HDL, Triglycerides]
- Waist size [cm], Weight [Kg] and Body Mass Index [BMI]
- Blood pressure [followed with 24 monitoring if clinic reading is high]
  For test explanations see "Diabetes Health Profile" on pages 8-10.

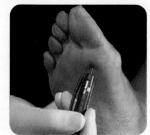

- Legs and feet examination to check your skin, circulation and nerve supply. If necessary, you will be referred to a state registered chiropodist/podiatrist.
- Eye examination where the pupils are dilated to enable the detection of any early changes at the back of the eye (the retina). Photographs are taken to record the appearance at the back of your eyes. The Department of Health has set up a National Screening Programme for Diabetic Retinopathy.
- If you're on insulin, your injection sites should be examined.

Eye Screening

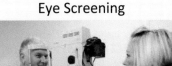

Diabetic eye screening is offered to all people with diabetes aged 12 and over every year. Screening is freely available on the NHS and is delivered by more than 80 local programmes in many locations, including GP surgeries, hospitals and optician practices. If you notice any new problems with your eyes between screening appointments you should contact your optometrist or your GP.

The things I need to work on to help look after my diabetes are:

My Cholesterol ☐

My Blood Glucose ☐

Tick if you have checked these in the last year and know what they are

My Blood Pressure ☐

Remember the importance of yearly checkups to your eyes and feet.

Tick if you have checked these in the last year

My Eyes ☐

My Feet ☐

Remember!!! 7 lifestyle factors that can help me look after my diabetes

- ○ My food choices
- ○ My weight
- ○ My alcohol intake
- ○ My medication
- ○ My physical activity
- ○ My smoking habits
- ○ My stress levels & sleep

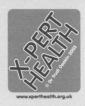

Further Information

If you have any questions about diabetic retinopathy:
- Ask your doctor or nurse
- Contact your local screening office
- visit http://www.retinalscreening.nhs.uk

Leaflets available:
- Your guide to diabetic eye screening [+ audio version]
- Diabetic retinopathy - the facts
- Preparing for laser treatment for diabetic retinopathy and maculopathy

Other websites to visit: www.diabetes.org.uk; www.rnib.org.uk

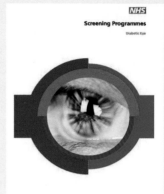

Your guide to diabetic eye screening

Lifestyle Issues

The annual review should also provide enough time to discuss:
- Your general wellbeing; how you are coping with your diabetes at home, work, school or college.
- Your current treatment (free prescriptions – if receiving diabetes medication).
- Your diabetes control, including your home monitoring results and hypos.
- Any concerns or problems you may be having.
- Smoking, alcohol consumption, stress, sexual problems, physical activity and dietary issues. You should feel free to raise any of these issues with your diabetes care team.
- The care you receive.

Having the right care is essential for the wellbeing of all people with diabetes. There is a minimum level of healthcare that every person with diabetes deserves and should expect. These are the **15 essential checks and services** you should receive. Download the checklist from the Diabetes UK website. If you aren't getting all the care you need, take this checklist to your diabetes healthcare team and discuss it with them.

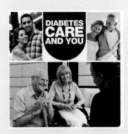

Diabetes Care and You [Free: Code 8010] and *15 Healthcare Essentials* [Free: Code 9863 available in several languages] available from Diabetes UK on 0800 585 088 or download from https://shop.diabetes.org.uk

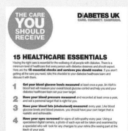

Depression and Diabetes The link between diabetes and depression is well known. Depression is very different from feelings of being fed up or sad. These feelings will usually pass as people learn and develop ways of dealing with them.

Depression is a serious condition which shouldn't be ignored and can be treated. It affects how you think and feel about things. It is not a sign of personal weakness or failure. You cannot simply 'pull yourself together'. Treatments include medication and counselling. Discuss the options with your healthcare team and together you can work out what is right for you.

More information:
http://www.diabetes.org.uk/Guide-to-diabetes/Healthy_lifestyle/Emotional_well-being/

Diabetes UK Careline can provide confidential support and information. The team are trained counsellors and can give you the time you need to talk things through. To speak to a counsellor call 0845 120 2960 9am–5pm, Monday–Friday or email: careline@diabetes.org.uk.

At Work

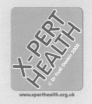

The **Equality Act 2010** protects people with disabilities from being treated differently to other employees. Diabetes is covered under the Act. If you feel you've been discriminated against because of your diabetes, then you may find this useful.

Further information: If you'd like further information, call 0808 800 0082 or visit the website http://www.equalityhumanrights.com. A *Diabetes and Employment* information leaflet is available to download from the Diabetes UK website at: https://shop.diabetes.org.uk/store/literature/booklets-and-leaflets/view-information-guides/employment-and-diabetes.aspx

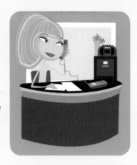

Driving

Recent changes to the Driver and Vehicle Licensing Agency (DVLA) medical standards will have a significant impact on drivers with diabetes treated with insulin (and in some cases sulphonylurea treatment). The most important change is that a Group 1 (car/motorcycle) or Group 2 driver (bus/lorry) who has had more than one episode of hypoglycaemia requiring assistance from another person at any time (including when sleeping) in a year, must inform the DVLA, and be advised not to drive.

What is a reportable hypoglycaemic episode?

Hypoglycaemia requiring assistance from another person day or night. This includes:
- admission to Accident and Emergency;
- treatment from paramedics;
- assistance from a partner/friend who has to administer glucagon or glucose;

It *does not* include another person offering or giving assistance where the person is aware of his/her hypoglycaemia and able to take appropriate action themselves.

If your diabetes is treated with insulin

Inform the DVLA. You will be asked to complete a form called DIAB1. You will then be granted a driving licence for upto 3 years. However, if you are experiencing hypos or diabetes complications to your eyes or legs/feet, the DVLA may request an assessment (DIAB3) by your GP/diabetes consultant. If the DVLA are concerned about your diabetes affecting your driving ability, they may withhold a licence or issue a 1 or 2 year driving licence. Don't drive if you have just started on insulin and your diabetes is not properly controlled.

If your diabetes is treated with diet/tablets

You do not need to inform the DVLA unless: you have had more than one hypo requiring the assistance of another person within the last 12 months; you begin to require treatment with

insulin; you have developed diabetes complications that have impaired your eyesight, your circulation and/or sensation in your legs; an existing medical condition deteriorates or you develop any other condition which may affect safe driving at any time in the future.

Managing hypoglycaemia

Having a hypo while you are in charge of a motor vehicle can be fatal. Don't drive if you have had more than one episode of severe hypoglycaemia in the last year or have difficulty recognising early symptoms.

Drivers treated with insulin should normally check their blood-glucose levels before driving and on long journeys at 2-hour intervals. Have a snack if 5 mmol/l or below and do not drive if below 4 mmol/l/. This may also be necessary for drivers taking certain diabetes tablets such as sulphonylureas. Ensure that a supply of quick-acting carbohydrate e.g. glucose tablets are always available in the vehicle. Avoid driving if a meal is delayed. If hypoglycaemia occurs, or warning signs develop:
- stop the vehicle in a safe place. Make it clear that you are no longer in charge of the car. Switch off the ignition and remove the key;
- eat or drink 15-20g of quick-acting carbs followed by a longer-lasting carbohydrate snack such as fruit or a sandwich;
- do not resume driving until 45 minutes after blood glucose has returned to normal as it takes this time for the brain to recover.

Carry ID indicating that you have diabetes. For people with impaired awareness, it is recommended not to drive without eating if the blood glucose is under 7mmol/l. **Further information**: The Department of Transport http://www.dft.gov.uk/dvla/medical/aag/D.aspx Diabetes UK at www.diabetes.org.uk/Guide-to-diabetes/Living_with_diabetes/Driving/. Alternatively phone the Diabetes UK Careline on Tel: 0845 120 2960

Insurance

Since the Disability Discrimination Act (1995) came into effect [now replaced with the Equality Act 2010], insurers can only refuse cover or charge more if they have evidence of increased risk. Challenge your insurer if you feel you are being discriminated against because of your diabetes. Notify Diabetes UK so that they can monitor the attitudes of different companies.

Inform your insurer immediately of your diabetes. At each renewal inform them of any changes in your condition or its treatment and ensure that the pre-existing medical conditions are not excluded in the small print.

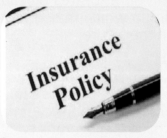

Allow yourself time to shop around to find suitable travel insurance. Sometimes it is worth talking to insurers before you decide your holiday destination. If you have complications, insurance for a trip to the USA could be much more expensive than other destinations.

As you approach retirement begin shopping around for annuities because some will offer a higher level of income than others.

Payment protection policies are normally offered to you if you take out a loan, mortgage or credit card. These policies are designed to help you meet commitments if you are unable to work due to illness or redundancy. Many policies will exclude claims for any medical conditions that existed prior to the start date of your policy, which could leave you unable to claim for any illness relating to diabetes.

Further information on diabetes and insurance: free download https://shop.diabetes.org.uk/store/literature/booklets-and-leaflets/view-information-guides/insurance-and-diabetes.aspx

For more details on Diabetes UK travel insurance visit www.diabetes.org.uk/How_we_help/Financial_services/Travel_insurance or call Tel: 0800 731 7431

DiABETES UK
CARE. CONNECT. CAMPAIGN.

Travel

- ○ Carry diabetes ID. If you are carrying insulin, a doctor's letter that explains your need for insulin and injection devices should be presented to the airline staff, as insulin should be packed in your hand luggage.

- ○ In addition to a doctor's letter, all adults aged 18 or over using insulin should have been given an Insulin Passport. This is so you can check you have been given the correct insulin and be able to show healthcare professionals which insulin and device you are using.

- ○ Plan to take twice the quantity of medical supplies you would normally use for your diabetes.

- ○ Make sure you have all your diabetes medication and equipment packed and take a list of the prescribed items in case they are lost and you need to obtain some more.

- ○ Remember to also include any other medication you are taking. Take a basic first aid kit with you especially if you are going off the beaten track.

- ○ If you are travelling across time zones you may need to adjust the timing of your medication.

- ○ If you are travelling to a hot or cold climate, this may affect how insulin works and you may need to monitor your blood glucose levels more frequently.

- ○ Your healthcare team can offer more advice about the vaccinations you need, timing of your medication and the impact the weather can have on you. Be sure to consult with them when planning your trip.

- ○ Make sure you have the European Health Insurance Card (EHIC) if you are travelling to a European Union member country - it will ensure that you have easy access to healthcare in that country.

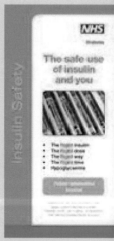

Travel

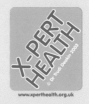

Find out more about the European Health Insurance Card http://www.nhs.uk/NHSEngland/Healthcareabroad/EHIC/Pages/about-the-ehic.aspx or obtain your EHIC from https://www.ehic.org.uk/Internet/startApplication.do. It is still advisable to buy travel insurance as the EHIC doesn't cover emergency return to the UK and not all countries give the level of cover equivalent to the NHS.

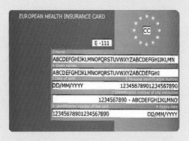

For practical information about the country you are visiting, Diabetes UK's wide range of country guides, with almost every country from Albania to Zambia, will also help you prepare for your trip. To order, please phone 0800 585 088, stating the country you wish to visit. For the latest information about the country you're visiting, including safety and visa requirements visit the Foreign & Commonwealth Office website:
https://www.gov.uk/government/organisations/foreign-commonwealth-office.

Further information: www.diabetes.org.uk/Guide-to-diabetes/Living_with_diabetes/Travel/

Sick Day Rules

○ Make sure you always have plenty of blood glucose or urine testing strips stored at home if these are relevant for your diabetes self-management.

○ Keep some basic medicines such as cough medicine and painkillers in the house. Make sure they have not passed their expiry date. Sugar-free versions are not necessary because you will only be taking them in small amounts.

○ If possible, make sure that there is someone who can help you out if you become ill.

○ Talk to your GP about possible vaccinations such as flu and pneumonia vaccine.

○ While you are ill, you may have to test your blood or urine more frequently.

○ Try to eat normal meals while you are ill. If you can't manage this, try regular snacks such as soup and sandwiches, toast or crackers, or milk and biscuits.

○ Nutritional drinks that contain a blend of vitamins, minerals, protein and carbohydrate can also be used if food intake is poor.

○ Increase your fluid intake to prevent dehydration. Drink at least 2-3 litres of sugar-free fluids a day.

○ If you really can't face food at all, take regular sips of sugary drinks – such as fruit juice or Lucozade – to provide you with some carbohydrate.

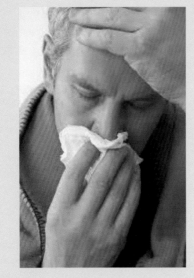

○ Contact your GP or healthcare team if you cannot keep down any food or liquid, or if you are in any way unsure what to eat or drink.

○ Keep taking your insulin or tablets to keep your blood glucose under control. The body's defence mechanism for fighting illness and infection involves increasing blood glucose levels.

○ Even a mild infection can cause blood glucose levels to rise. Your glucose tests may even show you need to increase your normal dosage of medication – if you are unsure about this, contact your GP or healthcare team.

rther information
tps://www.diabetes.org.uk/Guide-to-diabetes/Living_with_diabetes/Illness/

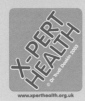

8 Steps to Diabetes Self – Management

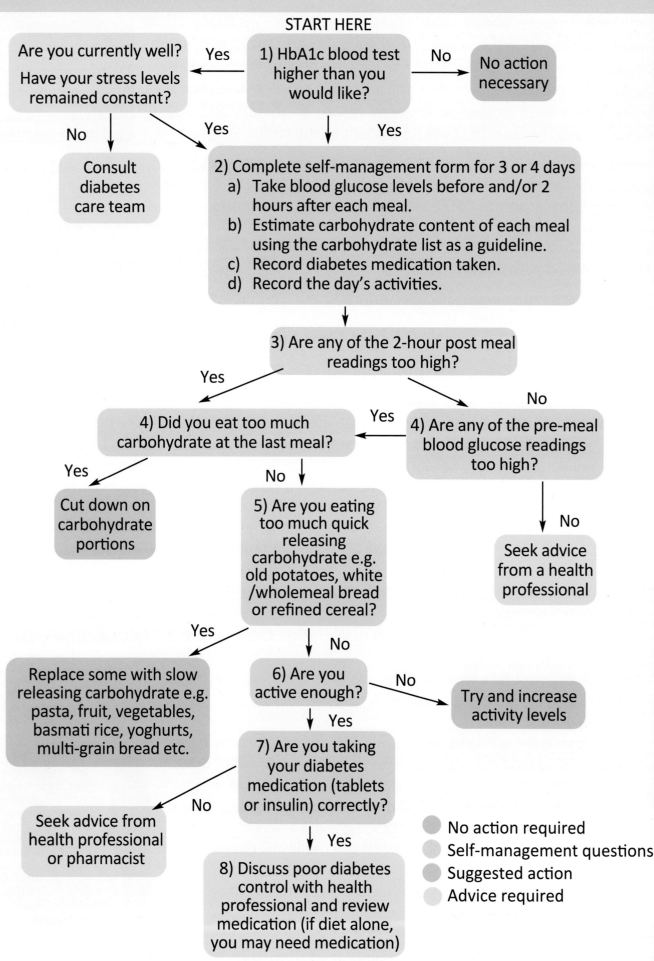

1) HbA1c blood test higher than you would like?

→ No → **No action necessary**

↓ Yes

Yes ← **Are you currently well? Have your stress levels remained constant?**

No ↓ → **Consult diabetes care team**

Yes → **2) Complete self-management form for 3 or 4 days**
  a) Take blood glucose levels before and/or 2 hours after each meal.
  b) Estimate carbohydrate content of each meal using the carbohydrate list as a guideline.
  c) Record diabetes medication taken.
  d) Record the day's activities.

↓

3) Are any of the 2-hour post meal readings too high?

Yes ← ↓ → No

4) Did you eat too much carbohydrate at the last meal? ← Yes ← **4) Are any of the pre-meal blood glucose readings too high?**

Yes ↓ → **Cut down on carbohydrate portions**

No ↓

No ↓ → **Seek advice from a health professional**

5) Are you eating too much quick releasing carbohydrate e.g. old potatoes, white /wholemeal bread or refined cereal?

Yes ← ↓ No

Replace some with slow releasing carbohydrate e.g. pasta, fruit, vegetables, basmati rice, yoghurts, multi-grain bread etc.

6) Are you active enough? → No → **Try and increase activity levels**

↓ Yes

7) Are you taking your diabetes medication (tablets or insulin) correctly?

No ← **Seek advice from health professional or pharmacist**

↓ Yes

8) Discuss poor diabetes control with health professional and review medication (if diet alone, you may need medication)

Legend:
- No action required
- Self-management questions
- Suggested action
- Advice required

Setting A Goal: Reducing Risk

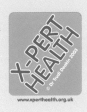

1. What is my biggest concern about possible complications of diabetes?

_____

_____

2. Why am I concerned and what would the benefits be from addressing the concern?

_____

_____

3. What steps could I take to tackle the concern?

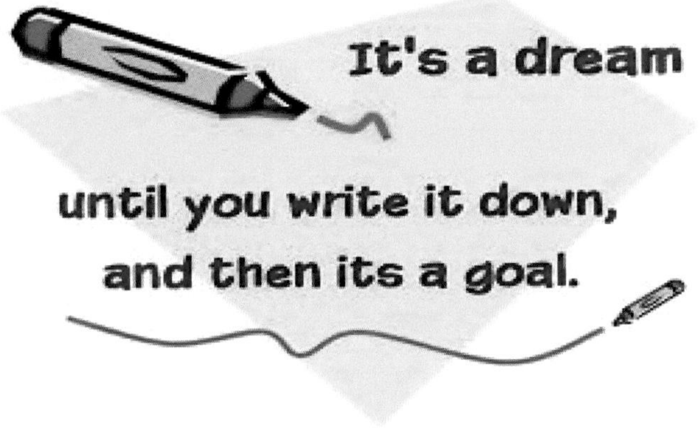

_____

_____

4. What is the first step I'm going to take?

What? _____

When?_____

Why? _____

It's a dream until you write it down, and then its a goal.

5. What happened? Did it work? How do I know?

_____

_____

How confident am I that I can make the first step? (circle)

0	1	2	3	4	5	6	7	8	9	10

not at all certain   totally certain

If you score below 7 - explore why ..... perhaps aim for a smaller goal!

Tick each day you achieve your goal and note comments

Monday   _____

Tuesday   _____

Wednesday _____

Thursday   _____

Friday   _____

Saturday   _____

Sunday   _____

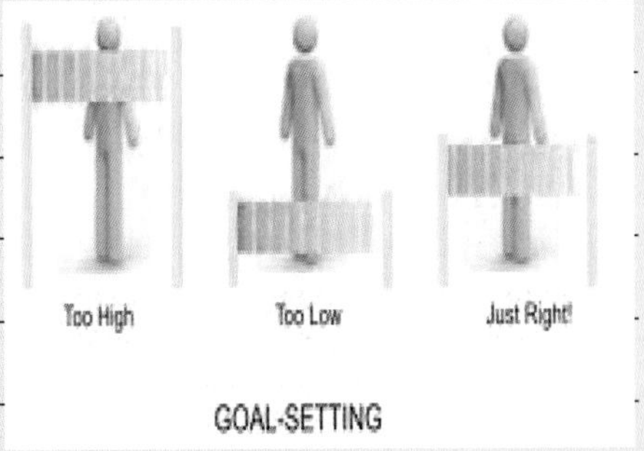

Too High   Too Low   Just Right!

GOAL-SETTING

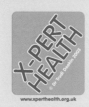

Section 6: Adapted Recipes for Healthy Eating

Fruity Tea Loaf

500g (1 lb) mixed dried fruit
450ml (¾ pint) strained tea
2 eggs, beaten
300g (10 oz) self-raising flour

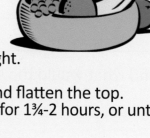

12 (98g) servings:
Per Serving
189 kcal
42.4g Carbohydrate
3.6g Fibre
1.1g Fat
18mg Sodium

1) Put the dried fruit in a bowl and stir in the tea.
2) Leave for at least 4 hours or preferably overnight.
3) Stir in eggs and flour.
4) Turn into a 1Kg (2lb) greased & lined loaf tin and flatten the top.
5) Bake in a preheated oven at 170°C/Gas Mark 3, for 1¾-2 hours, or until the skewer inserted into the centre of the loaf comes out clean.
6) Turn out of tin and cool on a wire rack.

Banana Nut Loaf

84g (3 oz) monounsaturated margarine
56g (2 oz) caster sugar
2 eggs
3 large ripe bananas (mashed)
112g (4 oz) chopped walnuts
168g (6½ oz) self-raising flour
56g (1½ oz) oatbran

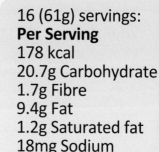

16 (61g) servings:
Per Serving
178 kcal
20.7g Carbohydrate
1.7g Fibre
9.4g Fat
1.2g Saturated fat
18mg Sodium

1. Put all the ingredients in a bowl and mix well.
2. Turn into a 1Kg (2lb) greased & lined loaf tin and flatten the top.
3. Bake in a preheated oven at 180°C/Gas Mark 4, for 1 – 1¼ hours, or until the skewer inserted into the centre of the loaf comes out clean.
4. Turn out of tin and cool on a wire rack. Slices may be wrapped and frozen individually.

Sweet Pinto Bean Tea Bread

84g (3 oz) pinto beans
200g (7 oz) self raising flour
½ teaspoon cinnamon
½ teaspoon mixed spice
56g (2 oz) monounsaturated margarine
56g (2 oz) dark brown sugar
84g (3 oz) golden syrup
1 egg, beaten
84g (3 oz) chopped walnuts

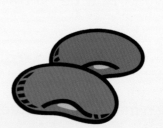

10 (61g) servings:
Per Serving
248 kcal
33.6g Carbohydrate
2.5g Fibre
10.3g Fat
1.2g Saturated fat
79mg Sodium

1. Soak pinto beans overnight, drain then boil for 1¼ - 1½ hours until tender; drain and mash.
2. Set oven to 180°C/Gas Mark 4. Grease and line a 450g (1lb) tin.
3. Sift dry ingredients into a bowl. Heat margarine, sugar and syrup until melted. Cool to lukewarm.
4. Add dry ingredients together with egg, beans and two thirds of nuts.
5. Spoon into tin. Sprinkle with rest of nuts & bake in a preheated oven.
6. Turn out of tin and cool on a wire rack.

Apricot Flapjack

100g (3½ oz) monounsaturated margarine
200g (7 oz) golden syrup
240g (8½ oz) porridge oats
100g (3½ oz) no-soak dried apricots, chopped

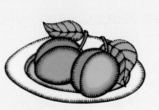

16 (40g) servings:
Per Serving
140 kcal
20.5g Carbohydrate
1.6g Fibre
6g Fat
1g Saturated fat
79mg Sodium

1. Lightly grease a shallow 18 x 28cm [7 x 11 inch] baking tin.
2. Melt the margarine and syrup together.
3. Add the oats and apricots, stir well to combine the ingredients.
4. Tip the mixture into the prepared tin and press out evenly.
5. Bake in the middle of a preheated oven (190°C/Gas Mark 5) for 20 minutes until golden.
6. Remove from the oven and leave to cool in the tin. Cut into 16 portions. Store in an airtight tin.

Adapted Recipes for Healthy Eating

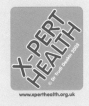

Date & Walnut Loaf

225g (8 oz) chopped dates
125g (4 oz) caster sugar
A pinch of salt
1 level teaspoon bicarbonate of soda
50g (2 oz) monounsaturated margarine
175 ml (6 fl oz) boiling water
1 egg (beaten)
50g (2 oz) chopped walnuts
225g (8 oz) self-raising flour

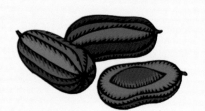

16 (57g) servings:
Per Serving
170 kcal
28.9g Carbohydrate
1.8g Fibre
5.4g Fat
0.7g Saturated fat
127mg Sodium

1. Place dates, sugar, salt, bicarbonate and margarine in mixing bowl with boiling water & mix until margarine has melted. Leave to cool.
2. Add egg, walnuts and flour. Mix to a batter.
3. Grease & line a 1Kg (2lb) loaf tin.
4. Bake in a preheated oven (170°C/Gas Mark 3) for approx. 1¼ hours or until the skewer inserted into the centre of the loaf comes out clean.
5. Turn out of tin and cool on a wire rack.

Chocolate Cake

225g (8 oz) caster sugar
4 eggs
140g (5 oz) self-raising flour
1 teaspoon baking powder
40g (1½ oz) oatbran
40g (1½ oz) cocoa powder
Topping: Sugar-free Chocolate Angel Delight made with ¼ pint skimmed milk

12 (53g) servings:
Per Serving
159 kcal
32.5g Carbohydrate
1.7g Fibre
2.3g Fat
0.8g Saturated fat
22mg Sodium

1) Beat together sugar & eggs until thick and frothy.
2) Add flour, baking powder, oatbran & cocoa and stir lightly with a metal spoon.
3) Spoon into a greased & lined cake tin and bake in a preheated oven (180°C/Gas Mark 4) for approximately 30 minutes (or until skewer inserted into the cake comes out clean).
4) Leave to cool. Cut in half and spread Angel Delight in the middle and on top of the cake.

Snack Bars

4 Weetabix™, crumbled
50g (2 oz) self-raising flour
75g (3 oz) no-soak dried apricots
50g (2 oz) sultanas
100g (3½ oz) pitted prunes
1 tablespoon rapeseed oil
1 large egg, lightly beaten
50g (2 oz) caster sugar
125 ml (4½ oz) low-fat natural yoghurt

10 (62g) servings:
Per Serving
126 kcal
24.2g Carbohydrate
1.9g Fibre
2.4g Fat
0.6g Saturated fat
13mg Sodium

1) Lightly grease a shallow 18 x 28cm [7 x 11 inch] rectangular baking tin.
2) Combine all the ingredients in a large bowl. Press into the tin and bake in a moderate preheated oven (180°C/Gas Mark 4) for about 30 minutes until golden brown.
3) Cut into bars while still warm but leave in the tin until cool. Store in an airtight tin.

N.B. Substituting sugar for artificial sweeteners that can be used in baking can reduce the carbs and calories per serving. Analyse your own recipes at:

http://caloriecount.about.com/cc/recipe_analysis.php

Diabetes UK recipes http://www.diabetes.org.uk/Guide-to-diabetes/Food_and_recipes/Recipes.

Cookery Books can be purchased at https://shop.diabetes.org.uk/store/literature/recipe-books

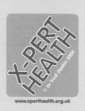

Understanding Your Medication

Medication to aid weight loss

There is currently one anti-obesity drug available on prescription in the UK. This has been shown to provide additional help to individuals when trying to lose weight.

	Orlistat (Xenical®)
Way it works:	Prevents the absorption of one-third of dietary fat
Prescribed for people:	Aged 18 to 75 years who are obese (BMI over 30kg/m^2] [BMI over 28 kg/m^2 with diabetes]
Special caution in people:	With digestion and/or bowel problems
Targets:	5% weight loss in 3 months 10% weight loss in 6 months But lower targets may be set for people with diabetes.

alli – this is an over the counter preparation of Orlistat at a reduced dose of 60 mgs. For more information ask your pharmacist or visit http://www.alli.co.uk

Diabetes Medications

Sulphonylureas

Taken once or twice daily with meals

These work by stimulating the cells in the pancreas to make more insulin. The dosage indicated will vary from person to person – if you have any problems with your dosage or frequency, contact your diabetes care team.

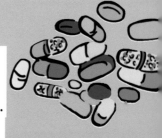

Name	Trade name	Initial daily dose	Min/max daily dose
Glibenclamide	Glibenclamide	2.5 mg, 5mg	2.5 - 15 mg
Gliclazide	Diamicron	40-80 mg	40 - 320 mg
Gliclazide	Diamicron® MR (modified release)	30 mg	30 -120 mg
Glipizide	Minodiab	2.5-5 mg	2.5 - 20 mg
Glimepiride	Amaryl	1 mg	1 - 6 mg
Tolbutamide	Tolbutamide	500mg	500 - 2000 mg

Side effects: nausea, stomach upsets, increase in weight. Very occasionally, a skin rash may appear If you have this contact your GP or diabetes care team for advice. Sulphonylureas can cause your blood glucose levels to fall too low, causing hypoglycaemia (hypo).

Diabetes Medications

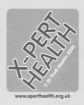

Biguanide

Taken up to three times daily with meals. This works in two ways. It helps to stop the liver producing new glucose and it overcomes insulin resistance by making insulin carry glucose into muscle and fat cells more effectively.

Name	Trade name	Initial daily dose	Min/max daily dose
Metformin	Glucamet, Glucophage	500mg, 850mg	500-3000 mg
Metformin	Glucophage Powder	500mg, 1000mg	500-3000 mg
Metformin	Metformin Oral Solution	500mg per 5ml	500-3000 mg
Metformin (prolonged release)	Glucophage SR Bolamyn SR	500mg,750mg, 1000mg	500-2000 mg (taken once or twice daily)

Side effects: upset stomach, including nausea and diarrhoea, which will often reduce with time especially if the tablets are taken with or immediately after food. To reduce side effects, doses should be titrated (increased) slowly.

Prandial glucose regulators

Taken up to three times daily before meals. These work by stimulating your pancreas to produce more insulin, but should only be taken at times when a meal is consumed. In this way they are shorter acting than sulphonylureas and therefore have a lower risk of hypoglycaemia. Flexible dosing can help to limit weight gain and people are less likely to require snacks between meals.

Name	Trade name	Initial daily dose	Min/max daily dose
Repaglinide	Prandin	0.5 mg	0.5 - 16 mg
Nateglinide	Starlix	60 mg	60 mg - 540 mg

Side effects: these can include upset stomach, nausea and skin rashes.

Thiazolidinediones (glitazones)

Taken once daily usually in the morning (twice daily for the combination with metformin). These overcome insulin resistance, enabling the body to use its own natural insulin more effectively. They also are available combined with Metformin.

Name	Trade name	Initial daily dose	Min/max daily dose
Pioglitazone	Actos	15mg or 30mg once daily	15mg to 45 mg once daily
Pioglitazone/ Metformin	Competact	15 mg/850mg twice daily	15mg/850mg twice daily

Side effects: these can include headaches, oedema (fluid retention), weight gain and less commonly upper respiratory tract infections.

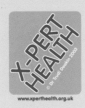

Diabetes Medications

Alpha glucosidase inhibitor (Acarbose/Glucobay)

Taken three times daily. It works by slowing down the absorption of starchy foods from the gut, thereby slowing the rise in blood glucose after meals. Initial dose 50mg, increased as tolerated to maximum of 600mg/day. **Side effects:** may cause wind, feeling of fullness or diarrhoea.

Sodium-Glucose Co-Transporter 2 (SGLT2) Inhibitor

This is a new class of medication which blocks the reabsorption of glucose in the kidneys and promotes excretion of excess glucose in the urine. It can be used in combination with other glucose-lowering agents including insulin.

Name	Trade name	Initial daily dose	Min/max daily dose
Dapagliflozin	Forxiga	10 mg once daily	10 mg

This is a new medication. Any side effects need to be reported to your diabetes care team. The clinical studies showed initial weight reduction seen with dapagliflozin was sustained.

Incretin Mimetic

Incretin mimetics mimic the glucose lowering action of naturally occurring gut hormones and are given by injections into the skin. They are prescribed in prefilled injection pens in different strengths. They reduce blood glucose levels and may also help with weight management. They can be used in combination with other medications. They work in four ways:

1. stimulating the cells in the pancreas to produce insulin in response to raised blood glucose levels;
2. reducing the release of glucagon from the liver following meals;
3. slowing down digestion, therefore glucose enters the blood more slowly;
4. promoting a feeling of fullness.

Name	Trade name	Initial daily dose	Min/max daily dose
Exenatide	Byetta	5µg twice a day by subcutaneous injections within 60 minutes prior to the two main meals of the day.	10µg/20µg
Exenatide	Bydureon	Bydureon is the same medical drug as Byetta, except Bydureon is slower released requiring one injection a week.	2 mg once weekly
Liraglutide	Victoza	0.6mg once a day, at any time but around the same time every day. Does not have to be taken with meals.	0.6mg-1.2mg [1.8mg in special circumstances]

Side effects: may cause mild to moderate nausea that will diminish with time.

DPP-4 Inhibitor

DPP-4 inhibitors "Gliptins" reduce the action of an enzyme that breaks down a naturally occurring gut hormone. This hormone helps to stimulate insulin production. People are less likely to experience weight gain with this medication. They can be combined with other medication but hypoglycaemia may be experienced when taken with a sulphonylurea or insulin.

Diabetes Medications / Insulin

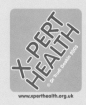

Name	Trade name	Initial daily dose	Min/max daily dose
Sitagliptin [Sita]	Januvia	100mg tablet with/without food	100mg tablet once daily
Sita + metformin	Janumet	50mg/1000mg twice daily	50mg/1000mg twice daily
Vildagliptin [Vilda]	Galvus	50mg once or twice daily. Can be taken with or without food	50-100mg once/twice daily
Vilda + metformin	Eucreas	50mg/850mg or 50mg/1000mg twice daily	50mg/1000mg twice daily
Saxagliptin	Onglyza	5mg taken with or without food	5mg once daily
Linagliptin [Lina]	Trajenta	5mg	5mg once daily
Lina + metformin	Jentadueto	2.5 mg/850 mg or 1000mg	twice daily

Possible side effects: headaches; inflammation of nose & throat; joint problems; painful extremities; respiratory tract infection.

Changing from tablets to insulin

Sometimes you need to start taking insulin instead of, or in addition to, the tablets you are taking. This means that your tablets are no longer able to control your diabetes on their own. Starting insulin injections does not mean that you have now developed Type 1 diabetes. You still have Type 2 diabetes but it is treated with insulin.

Once you have got over the initial fear of injecting [and most people manage this very quickly and wonder why they have 'put off' starting insulin for so long] you will hopefully feel very much better. Some of the symptoms of high blood glucose levels you may be experiencing will get better – you may feel less tired, less thirsty and will need to go to the loo less often once your blood glucose levels have improved.

The Range of Insulins

The information in the 'insulin section' is for general information only and will change as new insulins become available. If you have questions about any of these products, concerns about individual health matters or the treatment of your diabetes, please consult your diabetes care team.

Rapid-acting analogue insulin

Rapid-acting analogue insulin can be injected between 5 and 15 minutes before eating, when eating or immediately after eating. It can last for between two and five hours but, being very short-acting, it may not last quite long enough to control blood glucose levels between meals and may need to be used with a longer acting insulin. Rapid-acting insulin is clear. If you see 'frosting' around the bottle or particles in the insulin, do not use it.

Insulin type	Name of Insulin	Manufacturer	Vial cartridge or prefilled pen
Rapid-acting	Humalog	Lilly	Vial cartridge or prefilled pen
Rapid-acting	NovoRapid	Novo Nordisk	Vial cartridge or prefilled pen
Rapid-acting	Apidra	Sanofi-Aventis	Vial cartridge or prefilled pen

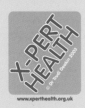

The Range of Insulins

Short-acting insulin

Short–acting, also known as soluble insulin, works quickly to lower your blood glucose and is usually taken 15 to 30 minutes before a meal to cover the rise in blood glucose that occurs after eating. It has its peak action within 2 to 6 hours after injecting and it can last for up to 8 hours. This insulin should always appear clear. If it is cloudy or lumpy, do not use it.

Insulin type	Name of Insulin	Manufacturer	Vial cartridge or prefilled pen
Short acting	Actrapid	Novo Nordisk	Vial
Short acting	Humulin S	Lilly	Vial, cartridge and prefilled pen
Short acting	Insuman Rapid	Sanofi-Aventis	Cartridge and prefilled pen

N.B. These are the most commonly prescribed, but there are others available

Medium/long-acting insulin

This insulin works over several hours to keep your blood glucose under control between meals. It usually has its peak activity between 4 and 12 hours after injecting and can last from 8 to 24 hours. It is often used in combination with short-acting insulin. This insulin usually looks cloudy. If the cloudiness is uneven, or you see lumps floating in the bottle, do not use.

Insulin type	Name of Insulin	Manufacturer	Vial, cartridge or prefilled pen
Medium-acting	Humulin I	Lilly	Vial, cartridge and prefilled pen
Medium-acting	Insulatard	Novo Nordisk	Vial, cartridge and prefilled pen
Medium-acting	Insuman Basal	Sanofi-Aventis	Vial, cartridge and prefilled pen

N.B. These are the most commonly prescribed, but there are others available

Long-acting analogue insulin

Long-acting analogue insulin is a form of long-acting insulin. However, it is different from other insulin because it is more slowly absorbed and therefore the effects of the dose last longer – around 24 hours in duration. It doesn't usually peak, therefore reduces the risk of getting a hypo. It is usually only taken once a day, in the evening. It is clear in appearance, as opposed to cloudy like other long-acting insulin. If any sediment is found in the insulin, it should not be used and should be discarded.

Insulin type	Name of Insulin	Manufacturer	Vial cartridge or prefilled pen
Long-acting analogue	Lantus	Sanofi-Aventis	Vial, cartridge or prefilled pen
Long-acting analogue	Levemir	Novo Nordisk	Cartridge or prefilled pen

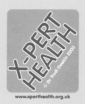

Mixed insulin

Mixed insulin contains rapid-acting or short-acting insulin mixed with medium-acting insulin

Insulin type	Name of Insulin	Manufacturer	Vial, cartridge or prefilled pen
Medium / Short 70% 30%	Humulin M3	Lilly	Vial, cartridge and prefilled pen
Medium / Short 70% 30%	Hypurin Porcine	Wockhardt UK	Vial, cartridge
Medium / Short 85% 15%	Insuman Comb 15	Sanofi-Aventis	Prefilled pen
Medium / Short 75% 25%	Insuman Comb 25	Sanofi-Aventis	Vial, cartridge and prefilled pen
Medium / Short 50% 50%	Insuman Comb 50	Sanofi-Aventis	Cartridge and prefilled pen

Analogue mixed insulin

Analogue mixed insulin contains both medium/long-acting insulin and rapid acting insulin.

Insulin type	Name of Insulin	Manufacturer	Vial, cartridge or prefilled pen
Medium / Rapid 70% 30%	NovoMix 30	Novo Nordisk	Cartridge and prefilled pen
Medium / Rapid 75% 25%	Humalog Mix 25	Lilly	Cartridge and prefilled pen
Medium / Rapid 50% 50%	Humalog Mix 50	Lilly	Cartridge and prefilled pen

Insulin pens available in the UK

If you have decided to use an insulin pen your choice may be determined by the insulin you have been prescribed. Alternatively, your diabetes care team may suggest an insulin pen that best suits your needs. Ask your diabetes care team for more information.

If you need more information you can contact:
Diabetes UK Careline: 0845 120 2960.
Open Monday to Friday 9am to 5pm or visit:
Diabetes UK website: www.diabetes.org.uk

NHS Direct Online:
www.nhsdirect.nhs.uk

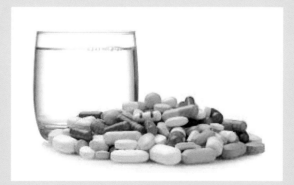

For information on individual treatments for diabetes visit the Medicines Guide website: http://www.medicines.org.uk/guides

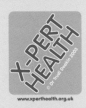

Blood Pressure Medication

Blood Pressure	Medications & their actions	Examples		Other benefits
People with diabetes may require up to 3 blood pressure medications	**Ace Inhibitor** (ends in ...pril). They allow blood vessels to widen & blood pressure to drop	Captopril Cilazapril Enalapril Fosinopril Imidapril Lisinopril	Moexipril Perindopril Quinapril Ramipril Trandolapril	Can delay the onset & progression of kidney damage. Available for people following a heart attack.
	Angiotensin-II receptor antagonists (ends in ...sartan) Similar to the Ace Inhibitor and may be used as an alternative.	Candesartan Eprosartan Losartan Irbesartan	Olmesartan Telmisartan Valsartan	They can help delay the onset and progression of kidney damage. They can also be used in the management of heart failure.
	Beta blocker (ends in ...olol / alol) They decrease the activity of the heart.	Acebutolol Atenolol Bisoprolol Celiprolol Metoprolol Nadolol	Nebivolol Oxprenolol Pindolol Propranolol Timolol	Used to treat abnormal heart beat and angina. Reduce risk of a further heart attack & heart failure.
	Calcium channel blocker (ends in pine/ mil / zem). Reduce strength of the heart beat, and cause the vessels to expand.	Amlodipine Diltiazem Isradipine Lacidipine	Lercanidipine Nicardipine Nifedipine Verapamil	They are used to treat angina.
	Thiazide Diuretics (ends with thiazide) increase volume of urine by promoting excretion of salts and water via the kidneys.	e.g. Bendroflumethiazide		A diuretic used in the treatment fluid retention, such as heart failure and oedema.
	Direct renin inhibitors inhibit the activity of renin and as a result, blood vessels relax and widen, making it easier for blood to flow through the vessels.	Aliskiren		This is the newest of the blood pressure medications and all side effects should be reported to your healthcare team.

Blood Cholesterol Medication

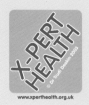

Blood Cholesterol	Medications & their actions	Examples	Other benefits
Blood Lipids • Total cholesterol • Bad (LDL) • Good (HDL) • Triglycerides	**Statins** (ends with statin). They interfere with the production of cholesterol in the liver.	Simvastatin Pravastatin Atorvastatin Rosvastatin Fluvastatin	Reduces the risk of cardiovascular disease.
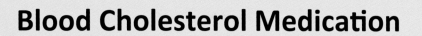	**Fibrates** increase the production of a chemical in the body which breaks up the cholesterol.	Bezafibrate Fenofibrate Gemfibrozil Ciprofibrate	Reduces the risk of cardiovascular disease.
Nicotinic Acid Deriavatives	**Nicotinic Acid Derivatives** reduce cholesterol and triglyceride levels (used in combination with statins).	Acipimox Nicotinic Acid	Reduces the risk of cardiovascular disease.
Cholesterol Absorption Inhibitors	Ezetimibe decreases cholesterol absorption in the gut. Can be prescribed with statins.	Ezetrol Inegy (Ezetimibe combined with Simvastatin)	Reduces the risk of cardiovascular disease.
	Omega-3-acid ethyl esters or **Omega-3-marine triglycerides.** Prescribed for people after a heart attack and to treat hypertriglyceridaemia (raised blood triglyceride levels).	Omacor Maxepa	Helps maintain supple and flexible joints. May keep heartbeat regular.
Other Medications	**Aspirin**	**Examples**	**Other Benefits**
Aspirin	Daily low dose of 75mg/day of aspirin is used in the prevention of blood clots. Helps thin the blood and reduce inflammation.	Aspirin	Reduces the risk of further heart attack, stroke or thrombosis. May help to reduce risk of developing cancer.

NHS NO...

Diabetes Health Profile

Traffic Light coding:
- ■ National target for good health
- ☐ Do I need to take action to improve my health?
- ■ What could I do to improve my health?

UK Diabetes Health Profile	*See pages 8-10 to for explanations. Below are the recommended ranges for good health. These are based on UK guidance from NICE* although your diabetes care team will work with you to decide what targets are best for you.	
Height (m)		
Weight (kg)		
BMI (kg/m²) weight for height measure	■ 18.5 to 24.9 = healthy ☐ 25 to 29.9 = overweight ■ More than 30 = obese	**Pre-Programme Results DATE:**
Waist Size (cm)	Men Women ■ Healthy - less than: 94 80 ☐ Increased risk: 94-102 80-88 ■ Greater risk - above: 102 88	
Blood Glucose (mmol/l)	Pre-meal: between 4 - 7 2 hrs after meal: less than 8.5 (T2) 9.0 (T1)	
HbA1c (mmol/mol) [Average blood glucose]	Normal: less than 6.3% or 45 mmol/mol ■ 6.5-7.0% or 48 to 53 mmol/mol ☐ 7.0-7.5% or 53 to 59 mmol/mol ■ Above 7.5% or 59 mmol/mol	
Blood Pressure** (mmHg)	■ Below 130/80 ☐ Below 140/80 ■ Above 140/80	
Total Cholesterol (mmol/l)	■ Less than 4.0 ☐ Less than 5.0	
HDL (mmol/l) (good cholesterol)	■ Men: 1.0 or above ■ Women: 1.2 or above	
LDL (mmol/l) (bad cholesterol)	■ Less than 2.0 ☐ Less than 3.0	
Triglycerides (mmol/l)	■ Less than 1.7 ☐ Less than 2.3	
Kidney Function: ACR eGFR	■ Men-less than 2.5 ■ Women-less than 3.5 ■ 60 or more ☐ 30 to 59 ■ Less than 30	
Prescribed Diabetes Medication	Type(s)	Dose

*National Institute for Health and Clinical Excellence **If you have Type 1 diabetes or there is any damage to the kidneys, eyes or blood vessels in the brain the national target for blood pressure is below 130/80.